Dementia with GRACE

A New, Positive Way of Dealing with Behaviors in People with Dementia, Second Edition

Vicky Noland Fitch, BSW/CDP

First Edition Published 2018

Second Edition Published 2021

COPYRIGHT © 2021 BY Vicky Noland Fitch

FLAMINGO IMAGE COPYRIGHT © 2018 BY Vicky Noland Fitch

All rights reserved. No part of this publication may be reproduced, distributed, or transmitted in any form by any means, including photocopying, recording, or other electronic methods without the prior written permission of the author, except in the case of brief quotations embodied in reviews and certain other noncommercial uses permitted by copyright law.

Edited by Kathleen B. Duncan

ISBN: 978-1-7372510-0-2

Dedicated to Etta

CONTENTS

Why You Should Read This 2nd Edition! i

Introduction v

Chapter One: Dementia Basics 1

    What is Dementia? 1

    Are Dementia and Alzheimer's the Same? 2

    Who Gets Dementia? 4

    When Does Dementia Develop? 4

    How Do You Know If It Is Dementia? 5

    How Is Dementia Treated? 6

    Where Do You Turn for Help? 7

Chapter Two: The Seven Stages of Dementia 9

    The Seven Stages of Dementia 9

    The FAST Scale 11

    My Observation on the Stages of Dementia 13

Chapter Three: Common Behavior Issues in Dementia 17

    Common "Problem" Behaviors 17

    Pacing/Wandering/Elopement 18

    Shadowing 20

    Sundowning 21

    Resisting or Refusing care 21

    False Accusations 21

    Agitation/Aggression/Striking Out at Caregivers 22

Chapter Four: Old Ways of Behavior Management 25

Chapter Five: Introduction to Always GRACE 27
    Terminology 28
Chapter Six: G for Gather Important Details 31
    How Well Do You Know Me? The Me I Used to Be… 31
    Why Does Knowing More About Me Matter? 32
    The Gather Tool 35
    Gather Tool Questions 37
    An Example of Needing a Gather Tool 40
Chapter Seven: R for Reminisce 43
    An Example of (R) Reminisce 44
Chapter Eight: R for Routine 47
    How Do I Establish a Routine? 48
    Sleep/Wake Cycle Disturbances and Sundowning 50
Chapter Nine: A for Always Assess and PIC'EM 53
    PIC'EM 53
    P: Pain 54
    I: Infection 55
    C: Constipation 57
    E: Environment 59
    Transfer Trauma 59
    M: Medications/Medication Change 62
    An Example of Why We Always (A)Assess First 64
    One Last Note About (A)Assess 66
    Sample Medication List 69
Chapter Ten: C for Calm 71
Chapter Eleven: E for Excite 75

Chapter Twelve: The GRACE New and Worsening Behavior Tool............77
   How to use the New or Worsening Behaviors Tool......................78
Chapter Thirteen: Examples of the GRACE System at Work...............95
   Pacing: Ralph..95
   Sundowning: Myrtle 99
   Pacing/Wandering which can lead to Elopement: Gertrude 104
   Shadowing: Juanita..108
   Refusing Care/Medicines: Olivia 112
Chapter Fourteen: Words of Wisdom 115
Chapter Fifteen: You Are a GREAT Caregiver!..121
One Last Word about GRACE 123
Notes 127
Appendix A: 10 Signs and Symptoms of Alzheimer's 131
Appendix B: Seven Stages of Dementia..133
Appendix C: Terminology and Abbreviations..135
Appendix D: GRACE 137
Appendix E: The GATHER Tool 139
Appendix F: Solution for Olivia..153
Appendix G: Sample Medication List..157
About the Author 159
Contact the Author...161

ACKNOWLEDGMENTS

I must acknowledge the geniuses in the "Dementia with Grace Caregiver Support Group" on Facebook. Their personal caregiver stories of struggles and of overcoming form the foundation of my online practice. What started as a forum for me to help them has blossomed into friendships, support, and a soft place to land for them and me. I owe a debt of gratitude to my flock.

To my editor, Kathleen B. Duncan: You have made this second edition sing. And you have made me show up for choir practice.

All my love and joy!
Vicky

Why You Should Read This 2nd Edition!

Are you dealing with "problem" behaviors as you struggle to care for your loved one with Alzheimer's or another form of dementia? If so, you are not alone.

Are you wondering why "problem" is in quotation marks? Well, read on!

I believe that although much is lost at each stage of dementia, there is much that remains. I believe that when you see the "why" of a behavior, it ceases to be a "problem" and instead becomes an opportunity for a deeper connection. Did you know some professionals (me included) believe most all behaviors are because of an unmet need? By understanding this basic tenet and then using that knowledge to reframe the disease and its effects, we can better meet the needs of those we love.

The techniques you will find in this guide will help you navigate the rough days and steer you toward more graceful days. This approach to behavior management has been developed over the years, working with people with dementia. In these pages, you will find a system for just about any behavior that emerges!

You will understand *how* to manage the behavior by learning *why* certain behaviors occur and what you can do to keep "problem" behaviors at a minimum. Using a proven, systematic approach to behavior management based on the acronym, **GRACE**, you will discover the meaning behind each step and learn how extending and receiving grace can help both your loved one receiving care and you, as a caregiver.

I will explain why certain behaviors occur and what to do about them in a straightforward, easy-to-find approach. This book is arranged so you can find a "problem" behavior and find a solution quickly. Still, I encourage you to start at the beginning so that you have a broader understanding of why the behavior began in the first place. Once you understand the system in context, it will make for less emergent behaviors overall. Let's get started!

Disclaimer - This book is a general guide only. It should never be a substitute for the skill, knowledge, and experience of a qualified medical professional dealing with the facts, circumstances, and symptoms of a particular case because each person's situation is unique. The author-publisher urge the reader to check with a qualified healthcare professional before using any procedure to assure its appropriateness. The author-publisher and their distributors are not responsible for any adverse effects resulting from using the information in this book. It is the reader's responsibility to consult a physician or other qualified health care professional regarding their person's care. The information provided intends to be helpful; however, there is no guarantee of results associated with the information provided.

Introduction

Second edition? Already? Yes! We are now three years into the first edition. Through one-on-one meetings, YouTube comments, book reviews, and countless conversations inside our Facebook Group, hundreds of situations have taught me more and more about the people I serve. I understand you better, and I cannot wait to add more knowledge to these pages. I also wanted to update the formatting. I want to always bring my best to you. So, let us start Edition Two right where we began the first edition: with muddy feet.

Why is there a flamingo on the cover of this book? Aren't swans the graceful creatures? Yes, and for a book that centers on grace, a swan might have been the most logical choice. But I like that flamingo. Let me tell you why.

Those glorious white swans with the glossy plumage, gliding across the water barely disturbing the surface, remind us that whatever furious paddling might be lurking below, all appear to be smooth sailing.

On the other hand, the flamingo stands webbed feet deep in muddy water shifting her weight from one leg to the other alternatively for reasons that are not yet fully understood. This shifting seems to somehow keep her perfectly balanced with hardly any muscle use at all. Knobby knees and skinny legs and a crooked beak and bright pink feathers suit her. She stands there, proud. Stunning. Colorful. Balanced. Just as elegant. Just as graceful. Even with mud on her feet. *Especially* with mud on her feet.

In my decades of working with family members with loved ones with dementia, what I see all too much are families who are trying to hold it all together on the surface, while underneath…in the home, in their hearts…there is a furious pace of "keeping it all together" while dealing with behaviors that are wearing them out and throwing them off balance. Because they are trying to be graceful swans, they would never allow you or me (or the neighbors or the church members or the family who lives out of town) to see them struggling. Never would they be seen with "mud on their feet." Trying for the umpteenth time to get Mama to bathe, or at least change out of the clothes she has worn three days in a row. Or trying to get Daddy to eat. (He has lost so much weight). Or dodging false accusations of stealing her things…or having an affair…or spending his money!! It is a solitary feeling. And like that swan, what is seen and what goes on behind the scenes is an entirely different reality. And if they ask for help, they are exposed someway…Will I be a failure? If I were a good daughter, I would know how to do this. If I were a *good* husband, I would never *think* of placing my wife in a Nursing Home.

I get it. Been there, done that. Although I have never had a family member with the disease, I have been in the trenches with hundreds of family members who have, slogging alongside them as we tried to find what works when nothing seems to work. When agitation and aggression, and stubbornness seem to be winning the battle. And, I have been there when it all just "clicks." Bathing is less of a chore. Accusations and agitation turn into amicable conversations. Wandering and pacing are replaced with meaningful activity. Visits flow.

In this book, I challenge you to see yourself as a caregiver for someone with dementia as a flamingo versus a swan. Yes, dementia has exposed you and your family to a new reality…and exposed your trial and error, successes, and failures. But you are still standing. Maybe on one leg, but you are standing! And seeking and learning and loving. This book will teach you how to regain your footing and enjoy your person with dementia as you help them through the stages of their journey. Your lives can be bright, beautiful, balanced.

After all, what do swans and flamingoes have in common? **GRACE**. Let's explore.

Chapter One: Dementia Basics

By the time you have picked up this book, you probably know the basics of dementia and need more specific information addressing the accompanying problematic behaviors. Be patient. We will focus on the behaviors that emerge due to these assaults on the brain in the coming chapters. But first, just to be sure, let's go over some basics.

What is Dementia?

My simple answer is this: dementia is an over-arching term that encompasses several types of diseases. Like cancer is an over-arching term wherein lies prostate cancer, ovarian cancer, colon cancer, etc. Dementia is a symptom of various kinds of neurological disorders: Alzheimer's being the most common type, followed by vascular dementia, Lewy-Body dementia, and so forth.

The more precise answer is that dementia is not a specific disease. It is a term that describes a wide range of *symptoms* associated with a decline in memory or other thinking skills severe enough to reduce a person's ability to perform everyday activities also known as Activities of Daily Living or ADLs. Most people think of dementia as just memory loss, but it is also function loss, impaired judgment, critical thinking, and reasoning abilities. I use the letters MCCJRI to help me remember the losses:

    M: Memory
    C: Concentration
    C: Critical Thinking
    J: Judgment
    R: Reasoning
    I: Insight

Personality changes are also common, as are impairment in vision, speech/communication, and comprehension. Because of the assault on certain parts of the brain, especially in Lewy-Body dementia, there can also be audio/visual hallucinations, paranoia, and delusions.

I refer to this assault as "The Broken Brain." You will read this and hear this on my YouTube channel, and in the group on Facebook. The diagnosis of dementia can be nebulous for some people. The "broken brain" is descriptive and is an immensely helpful visual. If you see someone with their leg or arm in a cast, you immediately know they have limitations on using the broken part of their body. Similarly, think of the person with dementia as having a "broken brain", and be reminded of the limitations of that part of them.

Are Dementia and Alzheimer's the Same?

This question is by far the most common question I am asked by the public when discovering I work with dementia. As mentioned above, several conditions cause **symptoms** of dementia: memory loss, loss of concentration, problems with critical thinking and problem solving, reasoning and judgment.

Think of it this way: dementia is a symptom (a result) of Alzheimer's like itching is a symptom (a result) of psoriasis. Dementia is a symptom (a result) of Lewy-Body disease. Itching is one symptom (a result) of renal failure. So, it is a characteristic.

It is usual to use dementia and Alzheimer's interchangeably, but it is not exactly right. You can use dementia in the abstract, but the correct use would be dementia of the Alzheimer's type. Or Lewy-Body Dementia. Or Parkinson's with dementia. The most common types of dementia are:

1. **Alzheimer's Disease**[1]**.** This is the most common type of dementia. I like to describe Alzheimer's as a slow process of going backwards in time. While it begins with short term memory loss (and thus, repeating oneself- because the person doesn't remember what has just happened or what they've just said), the person essentially goes back to earlier days, because the days of the present are no longer remembered. Long term memory remains strong while

short term memory evaporates. The process of Alzheimer's has been divided into 7 stages which begin with simple confusion and in later stages the person has lost significant abilities (to swallow, for example) and full-time care is needed. We will discuss this in the next Chapter.

2. **Lewy Body Dementia or Dementia with Lewy Bodies.** Lewy Body Dementia (LBD) is another common, yet frequently misdiagnosed or undiagnosed, type of dementia. A simplified explanation for what LBD looks like is that it is described as a combination of Parkinson's symptoms with Alzheimer's symptoms. The stiffness or rigidity typically associated with Parkinson's combines with the cognitive decline associated with Alzheimer's. In addition to these outward traits, one of the primary identifying factors of LBD is visual hallucinations. The hallucinations typically are of smaller people (children) or animals and are not always upsetting to the person with LBD. Problems with sleep patterns – waking throughout the night or the acting out of dreams are other identifying factors. People with Lewy Body also experience fluctuating cognition – meaning that they can have moments or periods of clarity and make complete sense – followed by other times of confusion and nonsensical thinking. Lewy Body Dementia causes its victims to be extremely sensitive to anti-psychotic medications which can typically help those with either Parkinson's or Alzheimer's. These medications can create potentially fatal conditions for those with LBD.

3. **Vascular Dementia.** This type of dementia – which is sometimes called "Post Stroke Dementia" is quite different from Alzheimer's or Lewy Body Dementia. Vascular Dementia is actually brain damage traced to cardiovascular problems, or mini strokes that caused bleeding or harm in the brain. The most outstanding symptoms that identify Vascular Dementia are when drastic changes occur immediately following a stroke. Changes can be in

personality, thinking or reasoning - all depending on the area of the brain that has been affected. Trouble with paying attention, organizing thoughts, or analyzing situations can all be symptoms of Vascular Dementia. So simply put, Vascular Dementia presents itself mostly through cognitive changes, which are the result of brain damage. The use of medications has been shown to prevent or slow further brain damage, therefore control the progress of Vascular Dementia.

Who Gets Dementia?

Dementia mostly affects older people, and the risk of dementia increases with increasing age. No, not every old person develops dementia, but the older you are, the more likely you are to be affected by it. However, please note, I have known several 100-year-old people with the mental acuity of a 20-year-old, and I am sure you have known older people with intact memory, judgement, and reasoning, too. Not everyone over a certain age is destined to have a dementia type, but the older you are, the higher your chance. These are guidelines.

Another common question: Is dementia hereditary? According to Professor Nick Fox, Honorary Consultant Neurologist at the Institute of Neurology in London with the Alzheimer's Society, "The majority of dementia is not inherited, but this depends very much on the particular cause of dementia. Some (rare) causes of dementia are very clearly 'inherited', for example, Huntington's disease...Some other dementias have both inherited and non-inherited forms. In the case of frontal-temporal dementias, 30 to 50 per cent of cases are inherited. Most cases of Alzheimer's disease are not inherited."[2]

When Does Dementia Develop?

Dementia is progressive, which means it starts out slowly and gradually gets worse over time. There are researchers who believe that Alzheimer's type dementia can be present for 10, 15, 20 years before any symptoms emerge.[3]

The initial losses are described succinctly by the Alzheimer's Association in a top ten list, "10 Signs and Symptoms of Alzheimer's."[4]

1. **Memory loss that disrupts daily life**
2. **Challenges in planning or solving problems.**
3. **Difficulty completing familiar tasks at home, at work, or at leisure.**
4. **Confusion with time or place**
5. **Trouble understanding visual images and spatial relationships.**
6. **New problems with words in speaking or writing**
7. **Misplacing things and losing the ability to retrace steps.**
8. **Decrease or poor judgement.**
9. **Withdrawal from work or social activities**
10. **Changes in mood and personality**

How Do You Know If It Is Dementia?

There are other issues that mimic these changes, specifically, depression and delirium, which come on quicker and are readily treatable and reversible. Depression can occur in anyone whether they have dementia or not. And some older adults develop depression whether or not they also have dementia. Dementia and depression can co-exist. Depression is defined as a loss of interest in daily activities and a general feeling of sadness. Depression is treatable and there are many meds which can help bring relief from this awful ordeal.

Delirium is defined as an acutely disturbed state of mind that occurs in fever, intoxication, and other disorders and is characterized by restlessness, illusions, and incoherence of thought and speech. Delirium usually is a result of an infection in people with dementia…particularly in UTI's (urinary tract infections). This can also coexist with dementia, and depression.

It is always advisable to seek medical attention immediately if you notice significant changes in mood, behavior, thinking or judgment. A trained medical doctor can rule out reversible conditions and begin a regimen to address these issues. If these causes are ruled out and dementia is then suspected, there are courses of treatment that can mitigate the effects of dementia in the early stages and improve the lives of sufferers.

How Is Dementia Treated?

A doctor will usually begin by taking a good family history if one is not already known. This maybe a simple checklist in her paperwork. Then she will perform a thorough physical exam along with lab work to rule out any common issues (like a Vit B-12 deficiency) which can be treated. As I just stated above, a UTI can cause delirium, which mimics dementia, so the doctor will need to rule out other issues. Then a mental status exam is performed, the exam will test the person's orientation, (person, place, time, situation) along with critical thinking skills, etc. She may refer the patient to a neurologists or neuropsychologist to perform detailed cognitive testing. If the doctor suspects dementia, other tests can be performed like lumbar puncture to assess cerebrospinal fluid for protein markers and/or an CT scan, MRI, etc. which can detect structural changes in the brain.

The doctor can then make a diagnosis: sometimes it is Mild Cognitive Impairment (MCI). This does *not* mean eventual dementia, but it could mean you caught dementia early.

I would encourage calm at this point. No matter what the diagnosis. If the dementia is farther advanced, and is stage 3 or 4, it can be managed by taking intentional steps to care for the person AND the following challenges.

You do not need to know a diagnosis or a stage. These techniques in this book work with all people, regardless of if they have an actual diagnosis.

What do I mean about "the stages"? I discuss this in the next chapter.

Where Do You Turn for Help?

There are countless numbers of excellent resources available about dementia, its causes, and effects, so I will not repeat all of that here. Instead, I will list my go-to resources.

The Alzheimer's Association – www.alz.org
Tons of information on all the basics, plus ways you can become involved.

National Institute on Aging
https://www.nia.nih.gov/health/alzheimers

National Association for Aging
The number one link that I share with caregivers that they don't know anything about is the National Association for Aging! The website is www.n4a.com. This is a national outreach program that supports the area agency on aging system in America. The area agency on aging is a clearinghouse of resources in the area in which you live. It is an invaluable resource for caregivers because it tells you about what's available in your local area.

If you are aware of the type of dementia you are dealing with, please Google that "*dementia name* Association" to find out more about that specific condition. For instance, if you type in "Lewy body Dementia Association" it will lead you to the Lewy Body Association, www.lbda.org

Chapter Two: The Seven Stages of Dementia

Much talk surrounds "What stage do you think my person is in?" or "My mother is stage 5." What does that mean?

There is a scale developed by Dr. Barry Reisberg which discusses the cognitive losses in Alzheimer's disease. Since it is far and away the most common type of dementia, the scale has been adopted across the board to speak of all dementias.

The Seven Stages of Dementia

The Seven Stages is vernacular for the Global Deterioration Scale, or GDS[5]. It is as follows:

Stage 1: No Impairment
During this stage, Alzheimer's is not detectable, and no memory problems or other symptoms of dementia are evident.

Stage 2: Very Mild Decline
The senior may notice minor memory problems or lose things around the house, although not to the point where the memory loss can easily be distinguished from normal age-related memory loss. The person will still do well on memory tests and the disease is unlikely to be detected by loved ones or physicians.

Stage 3: Mild Decline
At this stage, the family members and friends of the senior may begin to notice cognitive problems. Performance on memory tests is affected and physicians will be able to detect impaired cognitive function.

People in stage 3 will have difficulty in many areas including:
Finding the right word during conversations
Organizing and planning
Remembering names of new acquaintances
People with stage three Alzheimer's may also frequently lose personal possessions, including valuables.

Stage 4: Moderate Decline
In stage four of Alzheimer's, clear-cut symptoms of the disease are apparent. People with stage four of Alzheimer's:
Have difficulty with simple arithmetic.
Have poor short-term memory (may not recall what they ate for breakfast, for example)
Inability to manage finance and pay bills.
May forget details about their life histories.

Stage 5: Moderately Severe Decline
During the fifth stage of Alzheimer's, people begin to need help with many day-to-day activities. People in stage five of the disease may experience:
Difficulty dressing appropriately.
Inability to recall simple details about themselves such as their own phone number.
Significant confusion
On the other hand, people in stage five maintain functionality. They typically can still bathe and toilet independently. They also usually still know their family members and some detail about their personal histories, especially their childhood and youth.

Stage 6: Severe Decline
People with the sixth stage of Alzheimer's need constant supervision and frequently require professional care. Symptoms include:
Confusion or unawareness of environment and surroundings
Inability to recognize faces except for the closest friends and relatives.

Inability to remember most details of personal history.
Loss of bladder and bowel control
Major personality changes and potential behavior problems
The need for assistance with activities of daily living such as toileting and bathing
Wandering

Stage 7: Very Severe Decline
Stage seven is the final stage of Alzheimer's. Because the disease is a terminal illness, people in stage seven are nearing death. In stage seven of the disease, people lose the ability to communicate or respond to their environment. While they may still be able to utter words and phrases, they have no insight into their condition and need assistance with all activities of daily living. In the final stages of Alzheimer's, people may lose their ability to swallow.

Some doctors will discuss the stages as "Early, Middle and Late." The correlation is this:

Early = Stages 1, 2, 3
Middle = Stages 4, 5
Late = Stages 6, 7

The FAST Scale

When discussing the stages of dementia, we must include The FAST Scale[6], also by Reisberg. It discusses the Functional Losses, and is often used in Hospice care as a form of eligibility determination:

1   No difficulty, either subjectively or objectively.

2   Complains of forgetting location of objects. Subjective work difficulties.

3   Decreased job functioning evident to co-workers. Difficulty in traveling to new locations. Decreased organizational capacity.

4   Decreased ability to perform complex tasks, e.g., planning

dinner for guests, handling personal finances (such as forgetting to pay bills), difficulty marketing, etc.

5   Requires assistance in choosing proper clothing to wear for the day, season, or occasion, e.g., patient may wear the same clothing repeatedly, unless supervised.

6a Improperly putting on clothes without assistance or cueing (e.g., may put street clothes on overnight clothes, or put shoes on wrong feet, or have difficulty buttoning clothing) occasionally or more frequently over the past weeks.

6b Unable to bathe (shower) properly (e.g., difficulty adjusting bathwater (shower) temperature) occasionally or more frequently over the past weeks.

6c Inability to handle mechanics of toileting (e.g., forgets to flush the toilet, does not wipe properly or properly dispose of toilet tissue) occasionally or more frequently over the past weeks.

6d Urinary incontinence (occasionally or more frequently over the past weeks).

6e Fecal incontinence (occasionally or more frequently over the past weeks).

7a Ability to speak limited to approximately a half a dozen intelligible different words or fewer, in the course of an average day or in the course of an intensive interview.

7b Speech ability limited to the use of a single intelligible word in an average day or in the course of an interview (the person may repeat the word over and over).

7c Ambulatory ability lost (cannot walk without personal assistance).

7d Cannot sit up without assistance (e.g., the individual will fall over if there are no lateral rests [arms] on the chair).

7e Loss of ability to smile.

7f Loss of ability to hold up head independently.

My Observation on the Stages of Dementia

Now that I have given you the technical definition of the stages, let me share some of my observations:

Stage 1
This is merely a placeholder for when there was no dementia observed by the person with dementia or the people around them.

Stage 2
There may be some benign forgetfulness here. Loss of keys, wallet, or phone with eventual retrieval; forgetting where you parked your car temporarily or needing reminders about appointments. This is normal forgetfulness and if it stopped here, would be normal age-related cognition. It is annoying to the person with dementia, but it has not yet traveled into serious territory. The person would score in the normal range of cognitive functioning if tested.

Stage 3
At this stage, the person may still be functioning in their environment, even working, with lots of support from mnemonic devices, lists, calendars, alarms, etc. The person AND their family and colleagues can tell something is wrong. Word finding difficulties often appear. They can visually describe something, usually better than word recall. Fresh information seems to not register in the brain as a new memory. They may repeat themselves over and over. At this stage, they may lose valuables without being able to find them independently. They may have trouble navigating home, and the discussion of driving will surface.

Stage 4
I say that Stage 4 is "as bad as they will get while still knowing how bad they are." It is a rough stage for the person with dementia because they are acutely aware of their losses yet unable to do anything about them.

They can be defensive, depressed, or discouraged. If Stage Three didn't prompt a visit to a neurologist, Stage Four certainly will. Clear deficits will be revealed on cognitive testing. They will need help paying bills, taking medicine, and planning meals/grocery shopping. They will need thorough supervision if living alone, and the doctor and family should decide that.

Stage 5
Cognitive and functional abilities are clearly diminished here. The person with dementia often seems more satisfied, less troubled by their losses. They tend to follow "their person" around (Shadowing), ask questions repeatedly, get stuck on a task or thought (perseveration). They generally need 24-hour supervision here as they would forget their medicine or take it twice, for example. They need help with bathing and other hygiene tasks.

Stage 6
Functional losses here include both bladder and bowel incontinence. Cognitive losses include not remembering names of spouse, children. Will associate more and more with "Mama" and siblings, asking for those people versus the people now in their circle. That begins in Stage 5, deepens here.

Stage 7
This is a very infantile stage, with the person with dementia presenting in bed, as they are usually unable to walk, have a lack of torso control. There is limited interaction with caregivers.

These observations are a brief characterization of each stage.

I hope this information has been helpful. We must remember, the person with dementia is not *giving* us a hard time, they are *having* a hard time Their brain is broken. I talk about that reality often with caregivers who think the person is misbehaving on purpose. They are not. *They are having a hard time*. When you look at the whole person, and they are physically fine, remember their brain is not. Their brain is broken and simply cannot do the things you are asking of them because of that. So, show them some grace.

I would HIGHLY recommend going to my YouTube channel for virtual teaching about the Stages. Search "Dementia with Grace" and find the Playlist on Stages. https://bit.ly/3eLeUZ5

Chapter Three: Common Behavior Issues in Dementia

Common "Problem" Behaviors

When I worked exclusively in a long-term care facility and was the Director of a dementia unit – also known as a Memory Care Unit (MC) – the referrals that came my way from both inside the facility and from the community had generally one thing in common: a person with dementia had a behavior problem which could no longer be controlled in the environment in which they lived.

The most common types of behavior problems:

- Pacing/Wandering which can lead to Elopement.
- Shadowing
- Sundowning
- Resisting or Refusing care (Activities of Daily Living, or ADLs) such as bathing, changing clothes, eating, taking medicine
- False Accusations
- Agitation
- Aggression
- Striking Out at Caregivers

Wandering away from home or being an elopement risk at the facility were often the primary motivating factors that prompted a referral to the Memory Care Unit. At that point, there is a serious risk of personal injury and that behavior cannot be ignored.

The other behaviors are less dangerous initially but can cause chronic issues. Refusing to change clothes or bathe can become a hygiene issue and lead to skin breakdown, for instance. False accusations, agitation, and aggression can cause severe disruption in a person's relationships, leading to fights with others, skin tears from striking out, and falls. These behaviors occurring concurrently or, individually if severe enough, would also trigger a referral to MC.

Let's talk about each behavior individually. I will begin by defining what each behavior is and how it *usually* manifests. These may look different in your person, but there are some general traits common to each. Some of these behaviors are problems for the person with dementia, and some are problems for people in their environment, which, in turn, creates problems for the person. Next, I will describe the impetus of each. As I stated in the introduction, I firmly believe that almost all behaviors are because of an UNMET NEED. I have found in my practice that when you meet the need, you solve the problem. We will discuss specific ways to manage these behaviors in later chapters based on the **Always GRACE** model, but first I think it is important to set a foundation of knowledge on which we can then build. I challenge you to evaluate each behavior with that lens of "What does the person *need*?" It's an important frame of reference. Let's dig in.

Pacing/Wandering/Elopement

Pacing is a behavior that finds the person in constant motion. Sometimes in a linear fashion, going from one point to another without stopping, but more commonly in a sauntering, meandering manner. The person is usually easily distracted by the TV, or something they stop to putter with on a table. They may pace for a bit, sit to rest, and begin the pacing all over again in just a few minutes. Usually, people with this behavior have generally always been a "busy" person. They don't like to sit still, generally. It is not a problem for the person, to my mind, but in private homes and facilities where the person is constantly on the move, it can be unnerving to family members, or to other residents in facilities. What is the **need** ? To be active, to feel useful, to be engaged.

Wandering is similar to pacing, with the added motivation of an end goal. To go home, to go to work, to go to a perceived appointment. The person is fixated on going somewhere and can sometimes even articulate where they are headed. "I've enjoyed visiting but I must get home" …but they are home. There is a disconnect between their perception and reality. The intensity of the behavior is in direct correlation to the perceived impediment to their desire to *go*. If you try a reason with them, and say "You are home," most likely you will escalate that behavior to an argument, agitation, or aggression. What is the ***need?*** To be in control of their decisions (autonomy); to find a place they feel familiar; or to change their environment.

Elopement is a natural progression from wandering if the person is not in a secure environment. It is simply, "Getting out and getting lost." Because they have the motivation to *go*, but lack the executive functions of planning, reasoning, and judgment, they are at risk for wandering off into an unsafe situation and not knowing how to get back to safety. We unfortunately hear of this all the time in the news, and elopement can have dire consequences. The need is similar to that of basic wandering: self-determination and looking for something familiar. This behavior is profoundly serious, and, without necessary safety measures, it can be deadly.

Let me stop and say this: If your person is wandering even some of the time, you need to take immediate steps to secure their environment. Door locks, child safety doorknob covers, and other devices can impede the person with poor judgement and reasoning from leaving a safe environment and should be employed. Facilities use advanced door locks and keypads to secure their units. These are security systems to ensure the safety of people with dementia. Many systems can be found on Amazon through a simple search. My group has road tested many of these devices, and the ones they recommend are all available in my Amazon Storefront: Amazon.com/shop/DementiawithGrace. Do your research and find what works best for your home.

Of at least equal importance is to have a medical ID bracelet made which lists their name, a contact phone number, and their memory impairment. There are also safe haven type programs in most counties and municipalities who provide GPS devices to assist in a safe return of your person should they wander off. A quick Google search should help you find something in your area. Also, the Alzheimer's Association has an option for persons with dementia, from their website:

> Medic Alert® + Alzheimer's Association Safe Return® is a 24-hour nationwide emergency response service for individuals with Alzheimer's or a related dementia who wander or have a medical emergency. We provide 24-hour assistance, no matter when or where the person is reported missing.[7]

Now, I have had some people say, "Well, we don't want to restrict her movement" or "we don't want to take away his freedom." To which I say, "Would you put a barely crawling toddler at the top of the stairs and expect them to be safe?" No. Because the baby does not yet have the reasoning and judgement to differentiate between what is safe and what is unsafe. You must use substitutive judgement. Same thing. It *feels* different for our elderly family members because it feels like we are "telling them what to do" or "Taking away their freedom." What we must realize is that, like the baby who has *not developed judgement skills* yet, the person with dementia has *lost* those skills. It is our RESPONSIBILITY to keep them safe. No guilt, then. Do what is safe for your loved one.

Shadowing

Shadowing is the behavior in which a person follows another person around. Everywhere. All the time! It is usually the primary caregiver within the home or in a facility. In a skilled nursing facility, the person with dementia may follow another resident around. Usually, the "followee" seems to be in charge somehow. It can be annoying, to say the least, to a family caregiver who never gets a break from the constant intrusion. It can cause sufficient irritation to a fellow resident in a facility that the person with dementia is the recipient of a hearty, "Leave me alone!" which is demoralizing. We humans tend to guard our personal space very closely, and this constant invasion is unsettling. Therefore, it can become a problem for the person with dementia because it is irritating to the family or fellow residents in a facility. It causes disruption. What is the *need*? To be close to a person in authority. To be safe.

Sundowning

Sundowning is a late afternoon phenomenon which presents in the middle stages in some patients, not all. It is sometimes present in those persons and sometimes not. It is generally presenting as increased agitation, restlessness, moodiness, and overall worsening confusion. There are several theories about why it occurs in the late afternoon, as the sun is going down (hence the name), and most seem to believe it has much to do with the body's internal clock. It is very disruptive to the person themselves, and to the people in their environment. The unmet need? It seems to be *less* due to an unmet *emotional* need, than to a *physical need* for regulation of their body clock, which can be addressed by routine. We will discuss this further in the chapter on Routines.

Resisting or Refusing care

Resisting care is the act of not wanting to do something like bathe, change clothes, take medications, or eat. They make excuses or try to put off the activity until later. Refusing care, then, is the outright refusal to do a thing. Because taking medications is important to a person's overall health, as is eating or personal hygiene. It is deemed a problem behavior because it has a negative outcome. The *need?* Autonomy and self-determination. No one likes to be told what to do and when (or how) to do it. Toddlers don't, teenagers don't, and people with dementia don't! But there is a work around! Keep reading!

False Accusations

False Accusations are generally secondary to paranoia. Paranoia is a suspicion or fear associated with a perceived fact. Misperceptions happen usually because of one of two things: Delusions or Hallucinations.

A delusion is a fixed, false belief. They can believe false things about themselves, i.e.: "I am the governor" or "I own this building and I am going to fire all of you!" OR they can believe false situations: "I am being held against my will" or "I am being poisoned." Really any manner of things. The common denominator is that the belief is *false*, and it is *fixed*.

Whereas a delusion is a false belief, a hallucination is a false perception. Auditory hallucinations happen when a person *hears* something that is not real. Usually hearing disembodied voices or whispering is the most common experience. It CAN be pleasant to the person (waves crashing on a shore), but most times it is disturbing. They often hear someone plotting against them, or making fun of them, or some other distressing expression. Visual hallucinations happen when a person *sees* something that is not real. Again, this CAN be pleasant, they may also see a beach, for instance; but generally, it is disturbing.

Each of these things – delusions, and auditory or visual hallucinations – are acutely disruptive to the person with dementia, and they often lead to the false accusations: "You stole my billfold" when in fact he has misplaced it; or "I saw that woman come out of our bedroom. Are you having an affair with her??" when you know that no one else is in the house.

A firmly held belief or perception is impossible to reason away in the person with dementia, because the reasoning center of their brain is damaged. Therefore, trying to argue with or reason with a person with dementia is useless. Distraction is the best way to interrupt this behavior loop as it happens, but it is usually recurring. This is one behavior in which medication can be useful, but caution is advised. We will talk more about interventions in later chapters. The immediate **need** here? Comfort and reassurance.

Agitation/Aggression/Striking Out at Caregivers

I am combining this section because these usually piggyback off one another. Agitation generally stems from an overwhelming feeling of frustration that leads to anger. Agitation can then turn into verbal aggression, "I hate you!", "I am going to slap you", or "I am going to turn this table over!!" which can then lead to the actual physical aggression of acting out against physical objects (throwing chairs) or violence toward the caregiver. This commonly referred to a "catastrophic reaction." The need here usually begins as an expression of autonomy or independence. And not realizing that they may be making a poor decision, they fight (verbally or physically) the challenge to their independence.

Example: A person has not had a bath for four days (refusing care) and the caregiver knows proper hygiene requires that a bath must be accomplished. The person does not want to take a bath, lacks insight into the need, and again refuses. The caregiver insists. The person gets agitated. The caregiver approaches and attempts to undress the person in anticipation of the bath. The person becomes verbally aggressive: "If you touch me, I am going to knock the hell out of you!" and then the caregiver approaches and gets hit. Can you see the unmet need of self-rule and independence? So, what is the answer? He MUST get a bath, after all!!

What if I told you that you can learn how to meet these needs of freedom of choice, dignity, and self-expression, AND accomplish the bath? It's all about **Always GRACE**! Read on!

Chapter Four: Old Ways of Behavior Management

There are several schools of thought on ways managing behaviors. I have tried most of them. Most work with some measure of success, in varying degrees, with certain people. Some do not work at all. Some work for a while and then quit working. Believe me, I have experienced *much* trial and error! And I bet, by virtue of you reading this book, you have, too!

Two plus decades ago, when I first began my social work practice, the pervasive guidance for behavior management was "reality orientation." The thought was that if you could reorient a person to the present, you could reason with them and problem solve to reach a solution to whatever was agitating them. That worked with limited success because, what we now know, is that the judgment and reasoning centers in the brain are assaulted along with the memory centers. But we didn't know. Not then. But we were trying to figure it all out.

One episode vividly etched in my mind is that of "Ethel", a ninety something year old in our care. Again, this was way back in the early 1990's, at the beginning of my social work practice. Ethel was pacing the halls of the nursing home, crying uncontrollably, and the nurses could not redirect her. So, they called me. The new Social Worker. Fresh from Reality Orientation Training. I approached her as she was pushing against the locked door of the facility, sniffing and sobbing.

"What's wrong, Ethel?"

"I can't find my Mama." BIG SOBS

"Well, let's think about this. How old are you, now"?

"I don't know, maybe 80...or 90."

"Well, then, that would make your Mama pretty old, huh? Do you think she may be in Heaven?"

"Maybe so, because that's the only place I haven't looked". BIGGER SOBS

I shudder to even recall. I mean, pearl clutching despair that I could have ever even **suggested** that her dear mother was dead. That was THE LAST TIME I EVER used that kind of reasoning with a distraught resident. I knew there had to be a better way. Now I know to address the underlying need. In Ethel's case, it was for connection and comfort. I would reassure her that her mother is safe and loves her, then I would ask her questions about her mother. This would reinforce the soul connection she had with her mother.

Over the next several years I learned how to comfort, cajole, redirect, and reconnect with my residents with dementia. I have had failure and success, and along with the work and dedication of many esteemed colleagues from all disciplines and family tested and proven approaches I have discovered what seems to work:

Always GRACE.

Chapter Five: Introduction to Always GRACE

I know your reading time is limited, so I want to get right to the heart of the plan. I am going to discuss the "what is the plan" in this chapter, then take each step and break it down in the following chapters. At the end, I will give some illustrations of the most common behavior issues and demonstrate how you can use these steps to solve that dilemma. Ok? Great!

The acronym **GRACE** stands for:

(G) Gather Important Details

(R) Reminisce/Routine

(A) Assess (PIC'EM)

(C) Calm

(E) Excite

I developed this plan in response to needing a quick and memorable way to teach professional caregivers how best to understand and respond to behavior problems. When you are teaching in an assisted living facility (ALF) or a skilled nursing facility (SNF), time is of the essence. You need to communicate to a variety of disciplines…from housekeeping to dietary to certified nursing assistants (CNAs) to the Director of Nursing (DON) to the Administrator…a consistent way to work with folks suffering with memory loss. There are a lot of moving parts. You have different education levels, different responsibilities, different levels of interaction with the person with dementia. But each interaction needs to be consistent.

After teaching this method in facilities, I found that it could be just as impactful in the home. Some people with dementia do not need an ALF or SNF yet. Some decide to age in place with the help of HHC aides or private sitters. I had found something that worked, and I wanted to share it with anyone who would listen! Not everything works every time with everybody, but I have found this to be remarkably effective.

Some people never have a behavior episode, and some people have emergent behavior from the they time they wake up (if they ever went to sleep) to the time they stumble into bed.

This system provides a structure for everybody. It works whether behaviors are present or not because it sets up a routine to try to interrupt the behavior from ever occurring and provides remedies for when they do.

For the second edition, I added Always to Grace, because I use Assess first. And we are Always Assessing! We will discuss this concept more fully in the Assess chapter!

Terminology

A few notes about terminology and abbreviations here:

A ***behavior loop*** is my terminology for the beginning of a behavior problem to its natural end. At some point, left on their own, a person will act out and then calm down. At some point. An hour later? Two hours? And maybe after considerable damage to themselves or others, and certainly after a huge disruption to the routine in the home or facility.

Assisted living facility (ALF) is a type of housing – apartment, individual rooms, or shared quarters – designed for people who need various levels of assistance. Assistance may include medical or personal care.

Skilled nursing facility (SNF) is commonly referred to as a Nursing Home. Almost all are now known in professional settings and literature as a SNF. I began my career at a time when Nursing Homes were still referred to as just that. For that reason, I vacillate between terminology.

Certified nursing assistants (CNAs) are the caregivers who work directly with the person in an ALF or SNF. In the hospital or in-home health care, they may be referred to as ***personal care aides*** (PCAs). They are on the front lines in the care of the person. They usually have the best, first chance to avoid or interrupt a behavior loop.

You may notice I use person with dementia (PWD), "your person", and "loved one" interchangeably. I am aware that not everyone is taking care of someone they love because of various reasons. I try to be inclusive with this language.

A more complete list of terminology and abbreviations used when discussing dementia can be found in the Appendix.

Chapter Six: G for Gather Important Details

To meet the **needs of an individual**, you must know something about them **as an individual**. Not as part of a group (the elderly), not as a diagnosis (person with dementia), but rather as a singular and exceptional individual with a past. A rich history. A story of a life.

Every single person has a unique set of personality traits, wishes, wants, and desires. This does not change with dementia. These qualities may be affected by the disease process and its impact on the brain, but it does not diminish who they are, what they have accomplished, and what they still can contribute. Not only do they have a past from which we can learn, they have a present which can be refined, and a future which must be nurtured. There is always, always something to build on. In every stage, in a multitude of ways. By acknowledging and honoring the personhood of the individual, we can connect with the person, and thereby, manage the disease.

How Well Do You Know Me? The Me I Used to Be…

Genuinely knowing the person you are caring for is paramount for the kind of connection you will lean on to avoid, or to interrupt, a behavior loop. Now, in the home, you know your person. You may have been married to him for 60 years. Or she may be your mother and you have always been close and now, as you approach 57 years as her daughter, you think you know everything there is to know. But I have found that there is always more to learn, even for close family members.

For professional caregivers, whether they are in-home sitters, Home Health aides, or the staff of an ALF or a SNF, a full Life History is gold. They are learning the person for the first time.

At the beginning of my Social Work career in the nursing home, and really until my exit, a simple personal Social History was gathered on every resident. Straightforward, basic information was gathered to flesh out a person's social history. (A medical history was much more detailed. After all, they were coming into a nursing home, and the focus was more on the medical conditions to be managed). The social history is generally marital status, how many children, brothers/sisters, level of education...very general stuff, on a one or two-page form. Over time, the staff learned a good bit more about the person because we developed a relationship with the resident (person who lives in the facility). We began to learn their quirks and habits and routines which we then used to flesh out their plan of care. We learned if they preferred a morning bath or an evening bath, for example, and we used that to personalize their care.

Why Does Knowing More About Me Matter?

What I found when dealing with the people on my specialized dementia unit, the more I knew about a person, the easier it was to establish trust, authority, and understanding. For instance, I had a lady who would get really anxious around the 3pm shift change. She would pace and sometimes even try to leave the facility. From her simple Social History, I knew she was a nurse. I asked her daughter about her work, and she said she worked the 3p-11p shift her whole career. She loved that shift. What was leading to the anxiety at 3pm was the fact that she believed she was going to be late for work! She could see the other nurses leaving the facility and surmised that she should be part of the oncoming shift! Once we figured that out, we simply kept her busy with paperwork around that time (she wrote beautiful nurses notes based on data we provided about a "patient"), and away from the busyness of shift change. Loop interrupted.

Another man on the unit wanted to get under his bed on occasion and would become agitated if we discouraged that behavior. (Was it a problem, really? We will discuss that later!) Now, we had no idea what that was all about, and he could not explain it to us. A quick look at his Social History provided no clues. He was a retired factory worker. Father of three, widow. His children could not provide any insight either. On a visit from his brother, I described the obsession, and he provided the answer! The man had been a mechanic in the Army during WWII and worked under jeeps! His children did not know that fact about him. They knew he was in the Army, but not as a mechanic. We found a board with nuts and bolts and things on it, and that kept him busy with his hands. There are lots of options for things like this online. I have an Amazon "Storefront" that I will link in the Resources section of the book).

Behavior loops are not always about work. I consulted with a home on a lady who would hoard food and leave it in her bathroom. It became a problem because she was eating less of her food and hoarding the rest. She began losing weight, which can be a big problem. Plus, the food could not be left in the bathroom, for obvious reasons. However, when the staff would remove it, she would become so agitated that she fought whoever tried to remove the food. It was becoming a big problem. Talking to her daughter, we discovered that she was a Foster Parent once her own children were grown and had once fostered a child who was very thin when he came into her care. She was hoarding her food to "share" with this child, who was by now, a grown man and definitely NOT sleeping in her room, as her delusion led her to believe. The solution we discovered was to leave a "cleaned" plate in the bathroom with a note saying, "Thank you for the food, I am full as can be"! It worked. We could show her the note AND the plate if she started to refuse to eat (or to put food in her pockets), and she was satisfied that he had also been fed.

Now, these short paragraphs do not reveal the amount of work we went through to figure out the problem and devise a solution! Most times, it took us a while to figure it all out, and sometimes the first solution did not work. But with persistence and patience, we could usually solve the problem.

What I discovered, after both my work as the director of a dementia unit, and in the years that have followed as a consultant, is that the *groundwork* of a successful behavior management plan is a *robust, ever developing social history*. I call it a Life History. I created a questionnaire I call **"The Gather Tool"** with as many questions as I could fathom, using my own curiosity about a person's life history and questions found in various places online. As I discovered, it is ever evolving over the course of care. And I found that families who employed it as a tool in the home enjoyed the process of learning even MORE about their loved one!

Ready to explore this tool? Start on the next page and **(G)GATHER** some important details with The Gather Tool, or as some in the group call it, the Life History.

The Gather Tool

Instructions for Use:

Completing this Gather Tool is the first step in the GRACE Behavior Management System which is to "Gather Important Details." It sets the foundation of everything else to follow. These questions ask not only about the person here and now, but it also asks about their Life History. Know that the information you (G)Gather using this tool will be invaluable to making sure the other components of the GRACE system work. Knowing the answers to these questions will inform how you interact with the person with dementia. For instance, knowing a person's favorite type of music, and LEAST favorite, could help calm them OR engage them, depending on the behavior you are managing.

I would suggest reading through the questionnaire first to become familiar with the questions. Some might not be appropriate or needed. This is a good guide, but feel free to add or subtract from it as you see fit!

You will know best how to ask the questions to your loved one. Some people will welcome these questions exactly as they are presented here, with you jotting down the answers as you go. Some people would answer more readily if the questions were presented in a conversational style, a few at a time. Some loved ones would be VERY suspicious if you took out a pen and started writing down anything they said. Others would welcome the attention and focus on their lives.

It is a very personal exercise, and you should be respectful of their feelings, attitudes, and answers. If your loved one does not want to answer a particular question or delve deeper into a subject, respect that. Also, make a note of where an issue surfaced. That can be informative, too. For instance, if they are answering questions just fine, but clam up when military service is mentioned, that could indicate an underlying issue in that area. It might inform you not to bring up that subject again, or it may give insight into a behavior down the road. Similarly, highlight any information that makes a person "light up"! An area on which they could talk for hours! This will be your "go-to" topic to distract them if a behavior loop emerges!

All information, verbal and non-verbal, is helpful when dealing with someone with dementia. There will come a time when they are no longer able to answer these questions, and the information you gather while they ARE able will provide you a road map for when they are not.

Of note, if you are at a stage with your loved one where they are no longer able to answer these questions; use your own knowledge of their past to help flesh out the information or ask siblings or friends.

And lastly, have fun! Use these questions as a guideline. If a neat story comes up, go with it! You may learn more than you would have if you just skipped to the next question just for the sake of it! Engage in a conversation with your loved one; answer the questions yourself along with them! There is no right or wrong way to do this, so just jump in and see how it goes!

I am listing the questions here to familiarize yourself. The form with space to fill out the answers are both in the Appendix and available in the Files section of the Dementia with GRACE Caregivers Support Group on Facebook.

I suggest that this tool be kept with the person across the continuum of care. New caregivers or sitters in the home, temporary caregivers in a hospital setting, and caregivers in a new facility, should your loved one require that level of care. Of course, a copy of this book with how to use the tool and the supporting steps would be a useful resource, as well.

Here are the basic questions in the Gather Tool:

Gather Tool Questions

Name

- What is your full name? (First, Middle, Maiden, Last)
- Who named you?
- Were you named after anyone in particular? Why?
- Do you have any nicknames?
- Who gave you a nickname? Why? What does it stand for?
- Have you ever gone by any other names? Another married name? Another first name?
- What are you called by your spouse? Children? Grandchildren? Siblings?
- What do you prefer to be called?

Childhood Memories:

- Where were you born? What town/city/state?
- Were you born in a hospital? At home?
- Who were your parents? (Names)
- What did you call them? (Mama, Papa, Mother, Father)
- What kinds of jobs did they have?
- Did you have any brothers or sisters?
- What are their names?
- Did you have any nicknames for them?
- Are you the oldest, youngest? Where do you fit in the family?
- What is your earliest memory from childhood?
- Tell me about your home...
- Did you have any pets?
- Did you grow up in the city? On a farm? In a big place or small?
- Tell me about your neighborhood...
- Who were your best friends growing up? Tell me something about them...
- Where did you go to school?
- What was your favorite thing about school?

- What was your best subject? Worst subject?
- Tell me about your teachers...
- What did you want to be when you grew up?
- Did you have any role models or heroes as a child? Who did you look up to?
- What fascinated you as a child? What did you like to study or talk about? What new inventions did you like the most? Cars? Television? Space travel?
- Tell me how you spent your time as a child...

Adulthood:

- Were you ever married?
- Who did you marry?
- How did you meet your spouse?
- How did you propose/how were you proposed to?
- How long have you been married?
- Tell me about your wedding...
- Did you have any children?
- What are their names?
- Any grandchildren? Names...
- Tell me about your children...

Education and Work History:

- Did you go to school to study a trade?
- Did you go to university or college?
- Did you ever serve in the military?
- How did you decide what to do after high school?
- What was your first job?
- What was your main job or career in your life? Did you enjoy your work?
- Tell me what you liked most about your job? Least?

Hobbies:

- What do you like to do for fun?
- Do you like to play games? Read? Write? Draw? Sing? Cook?
- What do you like to read? Magazines? Fiction? Biographies? Religion?
- What are your favorite things to watch on TV?
- Any favorite movies?
- Where do you like to go on vacation?
- Tell me about some of your favorite vacations...
- What are some of your favorite foods? Least favorite?
- If you could travel anywhere in the world, where would you go?
- If you could talk to anyone in the world, who would you talk to?
- If money were no object, what would you buy?

Miscellaneous:

- Favorite color?
- Favorite song?
- Favorite actor?
- Favorite food?
- Favorite actress/actor?
- Favorite movie star?
- Favorite singer?
- Favorite type of music?
- Favorite car?
- Favorite place to spend time?

Can you see how knowing these things might help you care for a person with dementia?

An Example of Needing a Gather Tool

Below is an example of a situation where having a completed Gather Tool would have helped caregivers avoid what they considered "problem behaviors."

Marie was a 74-year-old woman who had been cared for by a sister who was no longer able to care for anyone, including herself. Her stepdaughter intervened and got help for both women. Marie ended up in the hospital severely malnourished and the sister went to a skilled nursing facility due to health issues. After a week in the hospital, two weeks in the Geriatric Psych Ward to establish a medication regimen, and eight weeks in an Alzheimer's Rehab unit, Marie was strong enough to move into an Assisted Living Facility. Her stepdaughter was not in town the day she moved into the ALF.

The first two weeks she was at the ALF, Marie refused to shower. Staff had tried many times. They had tried first thing in the morning, after breakfast, and the middle of the day. She wouldn't do it; Marie would not shower. They were also having trouble getting her to dress in the mornings and to bed in the evenings.

Marie's stepdaughter came to visit from out of state the second weekend after she moved into the ALF. The stepdaughter was able to get Marie to shower the first evening she was there. No problem. The next morning, Marie came out of her room fully dressed, hair curled, and make-up on at 7:30 ready for breakfast.

Marie's stepdaughter explained to the staff that her whole life Marie had showered and washed her hair every night before bed. Each morning she'd roll her hair with hot curlers (which her stepdaughter found in one of the boxes in Marie's closet). Marie wasn't "refusing the shower" any more than she was "refusing to go to bed." She just didn't want to shower in the middle of the day! Her stepdaughter told the staff she'd explained all of that to the folks at the Rehab Facility. The Rehab staff should have told the ALF staff. And Marie's curlers should have been in the bathroom, not in a box in her closet.

Having a completed Gather Tool which travels with a person from one facility to the next may help avoid issues like Marie "refusing a shower." Gathering this information will also help you establish trust, authority, and understanding.

In the Appendix you will find a copy of The Gather Tool which you can copy and use.

An expanded version of the Gather Tool is coming in summer of 2021. The workbook will be titled, "The GRACE Gather Tool (Expanded Edition)" and will be available for purchase through online bookstores.

Chapter Seven: R for Reminisce

Yes, this letter represents not one, but TWO words that we will use to help mitigate or manage difficult behaviors. One, **(R)ROUTINE**, is a given in the nursing home setting where I honed my philosophy and formulated strategies to serve folks with dementia. It will have its own chapter, next, but first let's **(R)REMINISCE**.

Let's dive in!

(R) REMINISCE is the natural progression to apply the knowledge gleaned from The Gather Tool. Having completed The Gather Tool, you now know a great deal about the person's Life History.

When people feel lost, helpless, confused…as loved ones with dementia often feel…they look for someone with the answers. Because our brains seem to constantly seek to create order out of chaos, it is only natural that if you don't know where you are, who you are, or any of the people around you, you want to find someone, **anyone**, who *does* know. It is our job as caregivers to be the person who knows the answers for the person who can no longer remember.

The DETA Brain Series[8] set of videos for professional caregivers proposed the following scenario: imagine waking up in a hotel in a foreign country where no one speaks your language, and you have no idea where you are. What would you do? Who would you try and find?

When I ask this question of people in my training sessions, they invariably answer "the police", or "someone in Authority!" Human beings are wired to seek out people with answers! And who has the answers? People who look like they are in authority, (which is why I insist on uniforms and badges for professional caregivers) or people who seem to *know* something about you!

Being KNOWN is being found. Being KNOWN feels like home.

If you are caring for a person with dementia in their home or yours, you probably don't wear a uniform, but you can let that person know that you *know* something about them. Talk to them about their past, tell stories you know of their childhood or early marriage, look through picture albums with them.

Knowing something about a person's Life History will help you care for that person. Knowing allows you to initiate conversation about something they used to do, prompt them to remember a story, or engage them in a hobby they loved when they were younger.

Knowing a person's Life History may also help you manage difficult behaviors. Sometimes a "problem behavior" is actually perfectly normal *if you only understood the person's Life History.*

An Example of (R) Reminisce

A friend sent me this example of how she used Gather and Reminisce to help a man who resided in the same Assisted Living Facility as her mom:

> John was a good looking, well-groomed man of about 80. He had a head full of silver hair. He always wore loafers, khaki slacks, a golf shirt, and jacket. The past three months I'd see him each time I came to town to spend a few days with Mom.
>
> (I live ten hours away so would visit 4-5 days each month. I'd stay in the facility's Guest Room. While there I'd eat with Mom in the dining room and participate in the activities. I was able to get to know some of the residents.)
>
> John constantly asked questions of the staff and was always getting in their way. He was often standing by the front door and would open it for any lady coming or going. When I arrived for my visit, he'd come out to the car, open the door for me, and offer to carry my suitcase. On sunny days he would walk along the sidewalk in front of the building.
>
> One day I noticed the staff becoming very frustrated with his incessant questions. Like many facilities they were short staffed;

they had too many things to do to sit and answer his questions! I, on the other hand, had plenty of time to talk to John. Mom was napping, and I was sitting in the common area reading and enjoying the fireplace. (Mom lived in a state with lots of snow and long winters!)

Having recently read "Dementia with Grace," I decided to try my hand at (G)Gathering information and (R)Reminiscing. Maybe I could help the staff by helping John. By helping the staff, I could ultimately make life better for my mom.

(I was not family nor staff so had no business trying to Assess him. The nursing staff would know if there were any urgent health issues.)

I engaged John in conversation and got him to sit with me on the couch, out of the way of staff. We chatted for more than hour. I learned the following:

- John grew up a military kid. His father taught him to "always be a gentleman."
- John was an Eagle Scout and believed in service to others.
- John lived in Florida (where he had a lovely garden) for four decades before moving here. He missed the sunshine and warm weather.
- John had worked in the prosecutor's office in a big city. He had been an investigator.

Aha! That's why he kept asking questions! He was investigating!

Mom had gotten up and I needed to spend time with her. But first, I asked John if he could help me by finding out exactly how many people lived in this building. He couldn't ask the staff, though; I was *investigating* them. He spent the next hour walking up and down the hallways on each floor counting the name plates on the residents' doors. Just before dinner he reported back to me that 57 people lived in that building. I told him he'd been extremely helpful.

A few days later, I met John's sister. She was there to move him to a new place.

The facility had decided he was "an elopement risk" because he kept leaving the building and opening car doors. They were requiring him to move to memory care, a locked facility, which happened to cost $1200 more per month.

His sister knew her brother and his Life History. She knew was not wandering or eloping. He just wanted to open doors and help carry heavy things for people because he was a gentleman. And on sunny days he wanted to soak in the sunshine and enjoy the gardens.

His sister was moving John to a Group Home where he would live with five other men who had cognitive issues. Round the clock caregivers helped these men live as independently as they could. And there was a big backyard with a garden where John could walk and enjoy the sunshine!

I was glad John's sister was doing what was best for John. And I was sorry the staff of that ALF had not read "Dementia with GRACE." They might have managed John differently if they had.

Because it would be virtually impossible for caregivers to keep all the answers to the Life History in their mind, it is important to highlight the part of the questionnaire that really "lights up" the person when asking the questions in The Gather Tool. These are the parts you can mention to a person searching for answers which immediately connect you to their story. It establishes trust and authority. It is amazing in practice.

I have approached people who were in the throes of a catastrophic reaction, mentioned a tidbit about their life, and, like magic, they calmed down and engaged me in conversation. Remember, almost all behavior is due to an unmet need. (John needed to investigate.) And what do we humans crave more than almost anything? Intimate connection with another. To know and be known. We can't fix the part of them that has lost the "I know", but we *can* connect to the part of them that says, "I am known." It is powerful.

Chapter Eight: R for Routine

(R) ROUTINE is simply the day-to-day actions that make up our lives. We get up, go to the bathroom, start the coffee, get the paper, etc. There are many variations of routine, but everybody has one. Everybody. It becomes second nature to us, and we don't think twice about our daily actions. Until they get interrupted for a few days.

Do you know that feeling between Christmas Day and New Year's? When you have taken that week off…your house is full of family home for a visit, you have eaten way too much and skipped exercising? You feel a little discombobulated, right? Consider this scenario: You kind of don't know what day it is when you first open your eyes, and you are not quite sure if you are off today or if you need to go into work; your sister woke up before you and made the coffee and is reading the paper. Your brother-in-law is already in the shower. And your wife is sleeping in. What do you do with yourself? It's an odd feeling!

For the millions of people with dementia, this can be their everyday experience. Every day is a new day, in a strange place…even though they may be in the same home they have lived in for 50 years. Some *things* may look familiar, but they may have lost who the people around them are. Or they may be in a nursing home where EVERYTHING is new, EVERY day.

What can ease the experience for them is (R)Routine. Something they can count on to use as a touchstone of familiarity.

Now, nursing home life is a (R)Routine in and of itself. Meals served each day at a set time, daily baths, medicine passes and a couple activities throughout the day make up a standard routine. But we go one step further with the people on our dementia units.

On the dementia units I have developed, we use a tight schedule of Daily Activities to keep the flow of the day on track. It is a deliberate schedule. There is something scheduled about every 30 minutes, and the same things happen at the same time every day. We have a printed schedule posted which is also printed as part of a newsletter that is distributed each morning.

The newsletter serves as a normalizing activity for the folks that received a daily paper at home, along with providing them a schedule. It features an article based "On This Day in History" OR a special commemorative day such as "National Ice Cream Day" and we plan the rest of the day around that theme. So naturally, on the Ice Cream Day, everyone gets a little ice cream as a snack!

All the daily activities in the morning are UP, UP, UP! Exercise is in the morning, group games are in the morning, Sing a long, Bingo, etc....morning time activities. After lunch, things start slowing down. Individual games and activities like puzzles, knitting/crocheting, watching a show about whatever the day is about (We celebrate a lot of what Elvis did on this Day in History, thus, we watch a lot of Elvis movies! Easy to follow and very entertaining!) We continue to slow down until bedtime, encouraging a natural flow of day to night.

I cannot overemphasize how valuable this has been. Even for the people who cannot tell time, or who cannot consistently tell time; they still find value in their printed schedule. One man kept his folded up and tucked in his hat!

How Do I Establish a Routine?

This could easily be replicated in the home, with or without a "newsletter", by using the daily paper, a discussion of the day's events and a set (R)Routine, not a set schedule.

This is one of the biggest changes to the second edition. I have learned that their (R)Routine trumps a schedule and is easier to maintain in the home.

Now, think of a set of monkey bars. Each part of the day is a rung. You swing through the bars gracefully, with an end in mind, and a good routine allows that smooth transition all day.

Rise and shine, grab a monkey bar, go to the bathroom, another monkey bar, eat breakfast...swing to the next monkey bar. Easy, right?

Every person's routine will be different. Some like an evening bath before bed (like Marie mentioned in Chapter Six), and that becomes a bedtime routine which can help with winding down and cuing that it is time to go to sleep. This helps with people who have trouble with their sleep/wake cycle...a common issue in folks with dementia.

Of note, everyone in the person's orbit should be on the same routine when interacting with the person. Writing down their routine will help assure that everyone is aware of it and can follow it.

It is best to have a schedule for caregivers coming in the home. Some people get one of those notebook organizers which have pages for the entire month and pages for individual weeks. The calendar/organizer can be open to show the month and left in a common area for easy access.

All appointments, outings, or regular events such as church are written on the calendar. The schedule for each caregiver, Personal Care Aide, or Therapist is also written down. Every caregiver can then see what is happening when.

Use the Weekly pages to document any changes in behavior or issues that come up.

Another good idea is to have a notebook to make notes of any changes. (The importance of journaling deserves its own book!) Amen!

If your loved one has lots of visits from family and friends, schedule appointments from Home Health Nurses and Therapist around family visits when you can. When you can't, explain to the family and the person who is coming and why. Tell them how long the appointment will last and assure your loved one they will have time to visit their family after the medical person leaves.

If your person rarely has visitors, perhaps it would be best to spread the visits from Therapist and the Home Health nurse over the days of the week so that they have visit one per day. Maybe have the Person Care Aide come on Monday and Thursday, the Speech Therapist on Wednesday, and the Home Health Nurse come on Friday. That way your loved one gets to see someone besides you almost every day!

Another note about (R)Routine, is the importance of (R)Routine places…having a "place" for everything is crucial, too. For instance, a member of our Facebook Group describes her person's dressing as this:

> "E always dresses by her bed. She has a safe place to sit and take off her shoes and the dirty laundry hamper is nearby. Her routine is to dress and undress in that spot. If she were to dress in the closet would be confusing." Plus, so many clothing choices in the closet would make it too distracting.

Sleep/Wake Cycle Disturbances and Sundowning

Let me stop here and make a statement about this issue. In some folks with dementia, there is a significant sleep/wake disturbance, and/or sundowning, which I discussed in Chapter Three They sometimes get their days and nights confused, which can be a big problem in the home of a family caregiver who works all day and needs to sleep interrupted at night. This is one of the main concerns I am asked about when I give talks to family caregivers. There is a part of the brain, the pineal gland, which is located deep down near the center, between the two hemispheres. Its primary function is to produce melatonin, which helps to regulate sleep/wake cycles.[9] It is affected by light, with darkness producing more melatonin (sleepy hormone) and light inhibiting that production. Nutshell: you need light in the daytime to keep you awake and darkness at night to bring on sleep. It is that simple, and that difficult.

In the homes of a lot of elderly people, with or without dementia, they keep the curtains and blinds closed all day. They do not venture outside in the daylight, primarily for fear of falling. They tend to doze off in a recliner in front of the TV. When night comes, they can't sleep. Sound familiar? Now, this does not describe everyone, but I would wager that if your loved one has a sleep issue, I have accurately described their day.

The way we address this lands right in line with the routine of the day. Once everyone is awake for the day, all the blinds are open, and the sunlight pours in! All the lamps and overhead lights should be on, providing for plenty of natural and artificial light to bathe the home. These activities and lighting are designed to wake them UP! After lunch start slowing things down. The activities slow, so turn the blinds to allow for dappled sunlight. Once supper is over, close the blinds and turn on lamps as task lighting, bringing the end of day literally into the home. It is amazing to observe the yawns, and the natural inclination to wander to their respective rooms and retire for the night. Now, you may still have some issues with sleep/wake disturbances, but it is much better. As the person progresses to the late stages, more sleep is expected and witnessed. So, allow for that!

If you do not have a set routine with your loved one, why don't you try it out? Start with establishing bedtime and wake time and try to be consistent. Even if your person does not get out of bed, open the curtains/blinds, and let the sunshine it! The pineal gland will do the rest!! Set mealtimes and a bathing schedule. It may take a little while to get a routine in place, but I believe, based on my experiences, it will be worth it.

Please Note: Because this is a (R)Routine, not a *schedule* , you start it at whatever time your person with dementia wakes up. If they had a long night packing to move out (very common), then when they arise, do things in the same order each day. As closely as closely as you can follow. Rung to rung to rung; it just starts

Chapter Nine: A for Always Assess and PIC'EM

I have named this A*lways* Assess! Because you are *always* assessing!

If you are a "hover mother" you recognize this phenomenon. It is where you are continually checking in with, and checking in on, your little one. Not a sniffle, not a bad feeling, not a scratch, not a tiny detail escapes your attention. Whereas this can be overkill in the raising of a child, it is paramount in the caregiving of a person with dementia! Let me explain.

Because a person with dementia cannot always express his needs or report important information or answer probing questions, the family or professional caregiver needs to be keenly attuned to those unexpressed needs, information, and answers! There are a few key issues that have the most impact in the life of a loved one...issues that can cause distress or discomfort or distraction...and if we are attentive to the five most common, it can make a huge difference in the quality of life of someone living with dementia. Attention to these issues, and addressing them proactively, can prevent a behavior BEFORE it even happens!

Since I have never met a mnemonic device I did not like, I created one to help caregivers constantly or Always **(A) ASSESS** their person:

PIC'EM.

> P: Pain
> I: Infection
> C: Constipation
> E: Environment
> M: Med Change

Let me explain each in detail. Once you know them, I promise, you will find them so helpful in day-to-day caregiving.

Note: It is vital when (A)Assessing a person that you TALK to the person. Ask them if they are in pain. Ask when their last bowel movement was. Ask them if something in the Environment is bothering them. Remember they may no longer be able to verbalize what is going on, but it is still important to talk with them, to communicate with them. Remember to treat them not a problem to be solved but as person to be cared for. While talking with them, WATCH and LOOK for no-verbal signs of Pain, Infection, Constipation, or Environmental Issues.

P: Pain

Whereas the *experience* of pain seems to vary in the person with dementia, based on several studies, the *expression* of pain is determinedly different. In the earlier stages, people are generally able to still express with some specificity their experience of pain: "boy, is my head hurting!" or "my arthritis is acting up" or "my elbow still hurts from where I bumped it." When they reach the middle stages, things get a little looser. They may hurt, but they no longer have the words to express the pain.

This is when non-verbal cues become so important. If they are rubbing their legs, knees, or shoulders, that can indicate painful joints. Constant repositioning can clue you into a general discomfort. And problem behaviors can emerge. Repetitive vocalizations are one such way that a person with dementia expresses pain or discomfort. Moaning or sing-song type of vocalizations may absolutely be an indicator of pain. But not everyone cries in response to pain. Some people shout out, some people grimace, some people winch. It is important to be aware of the baseline behavior so that if that baseline changes, it is a clue that something is off. There are some people who cry out constantly …it seems to be a self-soothing method…so someone who has that baseline behavior may not be in pain.

It is important to consider if they have a medical diagnosis that specifies there could be an underlying pain marker. Arthritis, degenerative joint disease, neuropathy, or history of any other painful diagnosis could clue you in to an unmet need of pain control. It is important to talk to the Primary Care Provider (PCP) to discuss ways to possibly provide for routine pain relief measures since the person with dementia is no longer to ask for a PRN (as needed) medication.

I listed PAIN first in my acronym because it can be immediately identified and treated, therefore, it should be the first thought when assessing a person's medical needs.

Non-Verbal indicators of Pain:

- a look of pain on the person's face
- hand movements that show distress
- guarding a particular body part or reluctance to move
- moaning with movement
- small range of movement or slow movement
- increased heart rate or blood pressure, or sweating
- restlessness
- crying or distress
- making more or fewer sounds
- withdrawing
- slowness to fall asleep or increased sleep
- disrupted or restless sleep
- low appetite (and consequently low nutritional intake)
- increased confusion
- anger, aggression, irritability, or agitation

I: Infection

Just as with pain, your loved one may not be able to detect an infection the way a person with a healthy brain can. And some infections may present differently in an older person than they would in a younger person. It is our job as caregivers to constantly be on the lookout for signs of infection, especially if new or worsening behaviors occur. It is part of Always Assessing.

It has been common knowledge for YEARS in the long-term care industry that one of the leading causes of a disruptive, new behavior in an otherwise docile person is a urinary tract infection, commonly referred to as a UTI. If a typically introverted, meek, graceful lady suddenly was crying, hollering, fighting or otherwise aggressive on my memory care unit, we alerted the PCP and he would order a UA C&S, almost invariably. (This is a lab test that checks for a urinary tract infection by culture and then tests for which antibiotic to which it is sensitive). It is standard operating procedure in most facilities with whom I work, because it is so predictive!

I do not know the statistics, so I cannot quote them here, but my GUESS is that when a new behavior emerges, and you have ruled out pain, infection is your culprit. Signs of infection always indicate a need for medical intervention. Call you PCP or Home Health Agency as soon as you notice symptoms so any needed tests may be done and medication started. Clearing up an infection will often cause the problem behaviors to resolve, though it may take time for your loved one to get back to their normal.

Non-Verbal indicators of Infection:

Indicators of possible Kidney/Urinary Tract Infections (UTI):

- Frequent urge to urinate (even if the person urinates very little)
- Pain during urination
- Cloudy, red, or strong-smelling urine
- Signs of pain in back, side, or lower abdomen
- Nausea or vomiting
- Mental confusion

Indicators of possible Ear, Nose, and Throat Infections

- Rubbing or pulling on nose, neck, or ears
- Tilting or waving head
- Red ears
- Trouble hearing – doesn't respond when called or talked to
- Holding, hitting, or banging head
- Refusing to swallow or eat
- Sounds different from usual (hoarse)

Other Symptoms of Infection

- Earache, fluid coming from the ears
- Sore throat
- Swollen tonsils or lymph nodes
- Bright red throat with white or yellow spots
- Headache
- Stuffy or runny nose
- Pain or pressure in face, tooth pain
- Reduced sense of taste or smell
- Fever

If there are any signs or symptoms of pain or infection, the Primary Care Provider should be contacted.

But what if it is not pain or infection? Next, please!

C: Constipation

People dismiss how important it is to have regular bowel movements. In facilities, everyone has a personal record of bowel movements, the size, and characteristics. It is either by self-report (the nurse or CNA asks about your regularity), or it is a daily report of the person who cares for your incontinence. Gross, huh? Intrusive? Maybe. But guess who else's bowel movements are CLOSELY scrutinized and reported to their primary caregiver? A baby. You know those little charts you get from the daycare about the dirty diapers? Same thing. A person's health can be assessed based on this very personal information. That is why it is so closely monitored.

Constipation can cause not only behaviors because of the physical discomfort it brings, it can cause an overall increase in confusion and irritability. I don't know about you (and I am NOT asking for a report!), but if I go for a few days without my "morning constitutional" I get so uncomfortable and moody! (I was taught that phrase by a sweet, graceful Southern lady as the way she described her daily BMs. Since I am a Southern lady, it is now my saying, too. You can borrow it. We won't mind!) If it happens to us, it can certainly happen to those we love.

Why does constipation happen? There can be many reasons. Slowed motility is an issue with the older generation, in general. Lack of exercise, multiple medications, poor diet...all can play a part. One of the most common reasons for constipation in dementia residents, however, is dehydration.

Dehydration is common in people with dementia because the thirst mechanism is affected. They simply don't feel thirst in the same way anymore, and therefore are less likely to ask for something to drink. I teach that if you are thirsty, offer your loved one a drink as well. Or set an alarm on your phone to offer them a cup of water each hour. Something routine.

Ever had to hear an older person talk about his bowel habits? Many older people are fixated about their BMs! Your person, however, may take offense at you asking about something so personal. You may need to get creative; you may have to use your nose to help you know if they have had a bowel movement. Just walk by the bathroom while they are in there. Or after they have come out of the bathroom.

This answer to solving constipation should be one of proactive measures vs. reactive measures. A little prune juice, some activity throughout the day, and a routine hydration schedule can help immensely. You may think about getting a small, lidded cup, something light and with a lid, to keep beside them during the day, as well.

Indicators of Constipation:

- Spending a lot of time on the toilet or in the bathroom without explanation
- Straining and grunting while attempting to pass stool
- Refusing to eat or drink
- Hard small and dry feces
- Hard, protruding abdomen
- Vomiting digested food that smells like feces
- Bloating and complaints of stomach discomfort.

If your loved one suffers from constipation and you are unable to resolve the issue in a day or two, contact your Primary Care Provider. Prolonged constipation can cause serious medical issues such as impacted bowels.

E: Environment

This letter of assessment means to evaluate the person with dementia's surroundings, level of comfort, and ease of being in a space. Any of these environmental cues could lead to a negative behavior.

Surroundings: Is it too hot or too cold? Is it too loud? Is it too crowded? Is it boring or drab? Or is it too busy? Are the lights too bright or too dim?

Level of comfort: Does the person look uncomfortable? Have they been sitting too long? Or walking too long? Are they pulling at their sleeves or trying to pull off their pants? Are they itching? Are their feet swollen making their shoes too tight?

Ease of being: Are they smiling or frowning? Do they look anxious or tense? Are they looking disagreeable toward a fellow resident or person in the family?

These are just a sample of questions to consider as you "hover" and assess. Train yourself to know the person's likes and dislikes, temperature (cold-natured or hot-natured), and overall way of being in the world. Then, if there are environmental stressors that run counter to that, you are more likely to pick up on distress quickly, and address needs before they turn into behaviors.

Transfer Trauma

One topic that comes up often in our Dementia with GRACE Caregiver Support Group is Transfer Trauma. Those asking about it don't know what it is called. All they know is that "Mama moved into an Assisted Living Facility about three weeks and now she seems to be depressed and doesn't want to do anything! She wanted to move there, but now she hates it! She is more confused, and her dementia seems to have gotten so much worse!" They are afraid it was a mistake to move Mama and don't know what to do.

What Mama is experiencing is called Transfer Trauma.

"Transfer Trauma" is a term used to describe the stress a person with dementia may experience when changing living environments such as moving from their home into a facility or from one facility to another. I am addressing it here because it fits with (E)Environment; the person's environment has changed, and the change may be causing new or worsening behaviors.

Transfer Trauma typically lasts six to eight weeks after a move or transfer to a now home or facility. During that time, the person may appear more confused, agitated, or even depressed. They may have more cognitive issues. Don't jump to the conclusion that you made a mistake or that medication needs to be added. These changes are usually temporary, and there are things you can do to help the person adjust.

One of the key ways to help a person with dementia overcome Transfer Trauma is to spend time with them before and after the move. Do what you can to help them adjust to idea of moving. Talk about what's going on. Explain about the move in terms they can understand. Of course, this may not be appropriate for everyone, but, if possible, let them be a part of choosing what goes in their new home, maybe even take them to see the new room prior to the move.

Once they have moved, write down their new address or room number in a prominent place where they can see it. Write out their new routine; print out the schedule for meals and activities. Show them where things are. Show them each and every time they ask where things are; don't respond with, "We already talked about this! You should know where things are by now!" Remember: their brain is broken! They need you to be a safe person who remember things *for them*. Walk with them to the dining room and eat with your loved one and other residents. Don't sit at a table by yourselves; socialize with other people. Escort your loved one to activities and participate in the activities with them. Do what you can to reassure them.

In some cases, it is best for family to stay away for a week or so to allow the person to settle in. Talk to the staff of the facility including the Director of Nursing, Social Worker, and Executive Director to get their advice. If you are not visiting the first week or so, be sure the staff are escorting them to the dining room and to activities. This is a common service given to new residents at most Long Term Care Facilities.

A few additional ideas to help with Transfer Trauma:

- When setting up their new room, place furniture and personal items as close as possible to the way the old room was.
- Get things unpacked and settled as quickly as possible. Don't expect them to be able to do it alone. They need help. Their brain is broken.
- Be sure to hang familiar art or family photos on the walls.
- Put some of their favorite knickknacks on display.
- Label things – Closet, Bathroom, Hallway, etc. – with large, visible signs.
- Stick with the familiar routine. Meals at the same times, same bedtime, showers on the same days/times, etc. Talk to the staff and inform them of this person's established routine and discuss how it will work in this new living environment. (A Gather Tool would be extremely helpful with this.)
- Ask them to escort her to activities and introduce her to new friends.
- If the move was into your home, limit outings and visitors until they've gotten more settled. Too many people coming and going may be confusing.

And get home health involved! Whether in an Assisted Living or a private home, Medicare will pay for home health for a person with dementia who has a new living environment. Many families have had physical therapy, occupational therapy, and speech therapy for weeks after such a move. The therapists do a wonderful job of helping people with dementia adjust to their new living environment. Plus, they can give you helpful ideas on making the move easier for your loved one.

Finally, be patient. The move is hard. On everyone. Give your person time to adjust. It takes six to eight weeks on average for a person with dementia to adjust to a new living environment. Don't jump to conclusions like her disease has progressed, she needs stronger meds, or this was a mistake. Change is hard. Give it time.

M: Medications/Medication Change

For reasons not fully understood, people with dementia are otherwise fairly healthy. The have fewer co-morbidities than their counterparts who share their decade. Because of this, they usually have fewer medications on board. Also, for reasons not fully understood, medications seem to affect them differently. They have more intense reactions to the medicines they need.

I learned from Dr. Richard Powers when starting medicines in this population we need to "start low and go slow", meaning start at the lowest dose recommended and SLOWLY titrate up, stopping when the side effects outweigh the benefits. This has proven to be exactly the right advice. The dementia populations I have served have been extremely sensitive to medication changes, and at times, seemed to act out worse when a new medication was added or increased. This is one area where, as they say, "Your mileage may vary," but I wanted to mention it as part of the area of "ongoing assessment."

If you have a new behavior manifesting in your person, and you have ruled out all the other PIC'EM measures, consider if a medication change may be the culprit. Has there been a medication change in the past two weeks? Some medications can take a week or two to influence a person. It may take time to build up in their system. Have you given them any over-the-counter medications for pain or allergies? Over the counter medications may interact with prescription meds. Always check with the pharmacist or PCP before giving dementia patient over-the-counter medications. Have any medications been discontinued? Has your loved one refused to take their medication or missed doses? These could all be causes of behavior changes.

You should always keep an up-to-date medication list. On your list, include:

- Medication name
- Brand name if it is a generic
- Dosage
- How often?
- When it is given (morning, noon, bedtime, as needed)
- What is it treating
- Date prescribed
- Prescriber
- Any special instructions.

Anytime your Primary Care Provider changes, adds, or discontinues a medication, you should update your list. Refer to this list when assessing your loved one. The list will help you know if any medication changes have happened in the past two weeks and may be causing this new behavior. I have included a sample Medication List at the end of this chapter.

Helpful hint: Keep a few copies of this Medication List so you can grab one anytime you are headed to a physician's office or when a Home Health Nurse comes to examine the patient.

An Example of Why We Always (A)Assess First

When new or worsening behaviors appear - although we do take a bit of time to quickly think about what we know from (G)Gather and (R)Reminisce and we look quickly at their (R)Routine - we don't spend much time on those steps until we have (A)Assessed the person. We (A)Assess the person using PIC'EM to check for any urgent medical needs. We ALWAYS do Assess first because it is most important.

(A)Assess is the center of GRACE.

Here is an example of how (A)Assessing a person quickly and completely can may a huge difference in managing difficult behaviors AND improve their quality of life:

> Sue lives in Idlewood Assisted Living. She is "pleasantly confused" per staff report. Her agitation started three days ago. She is now accusing staff of holding her hostage. She is demanding to talk to her attorney. Her daughter has reminded her that she chose this Assisted Living home herself after looking at several in the area. She chose this one because you can see the campus of the University from here, where she worked as an administrative secretary for over 30 years. Sue is not convinced by that reassurance. She is convinced that she was brought here just days ago, against her will. She is threatening to call the news agencies.
>
> The staff reports that Sue's thirst has changed. She is not drinking as much water as she had been. She excuses herself from activities to go to the bathroom in her room, and she has even had a couple of "accidents", which is unlike her. She smells strongly of urine, and the staff reports that her daughter will start providing adult diapers.
>
> Staff completed The Gather Tool upon her arrival. Nothing in her Life History indicates a history of paranoia. Her (R)Routine has not changed.

Sue needs to be (A)Assessed using PIC'EM as soon as possible to determine if there is a medical issue that is causing her new behaviors.

Remember, (A)Assess is the center of the system.

PICEM:

P: Pain
No Pain is reported, but staff notices Sue doesn't sit for very long, and she holds her back when walking. That is new.

I: Infection
When going through the Infection checklist, we noticed all of the following:
    Frequent urge to urinate
    Strong-smelling urine
    Signs of Pain in the back
    Mental Confusion

This sounds like classic UTI (Urinary Tract Infection) signs and symptoms. The doctor should be contacted for a workup (called a UA C&S: Urine Analysis, Culture and Sensitivity) to rule out a UTI.

C: Constipation
No sign or symptoms of constipation

E: Environment
No change to the environment

M: Medication Change
There have been no medication changes in the past two weeks.

If the UTI is determined to be the culprit, the prescribed medicine may cure the UTI. And curing the UTI should solve the behavior BUT can also cause other problems such as diarrhea or a yeast infection. The staff will need to be aware and on the lookout for any different complications from any new medicine added.

In this case, we have probably solved the underlying cause of the emergent behavior of false accusations, and GRACE has done its job. Because we (A)Assessed Sue at the beginning, we found a probable infection and were able to get medical intervention for her.

We can look to her (G)Gather Tool for ideas of how to (R)Reminisce and redirect her behavior until the infection is under control. Keep her on a strict (R)Routine - including regular bathroom breaks - to support her while she is being treated in house on an antibiotic therapy. It may take a few days, but her behavior should begin (C)Calm. There is no need for more (E)Excitement; there has been enough! Our focus is to calm her and reassure her that she is safe and loved.

One Last Note About (A)Assess

It is our job as caregivers to (A)Always Assess our person with dementia, even if they are living in a Long-Term Care Facility. We need to be on the lookout for issues which they can no longer see themselves. We cannot simply rely on the staff to take care of everything.

Here is an example one member of the "Dementia with GRACE Caregivers Support Group" on Facebook shared with me.

> Barbara was a dear friend to my mom who lived in an Assisted Living Facility. She was delightful! She was a widow with no children. Because she had no family and was no longer able to handle her own affairs, a Professional Guardian oversaw her healthcare and finances. I knew the Guardian because she had helped me a few years earlier when I was looking for a placement for my mom; we had stayed in touch.
>
> Barbara was an amputee who had a below-the-knee prosthetic leg. She was also a vegetarian.

One day I was visiting mom and noticed Barbara was in a wheelchair. She told me her stump had developed a sore that wasn't healing. She hoped to back walking again in no time.

Months later Barbara was still in the wheelchair.

I ate lunch and dinner that day with my mom. Lunch was a chef salad with ranch dressing. Yum! I noticed Barbara's salad had no eggs, no meat, no cheese, and no dressing. Dinner was beef stroganoff served over noodles. It was delicious! Barbara was served noodles. Plain noodles.

I called Barbara's Guardian the next day. I knew that due to confidentiality issues she could say nothing to me about Barbara, but I could tell her a thing or two. I told her, "Apparently the facility staff has no understanding of what "vegetarian" means. They simply removed any meat or dairy items from all meals served to Barbara. They were not providing protein in any other forms. No wonder her wound was not healing!"

The Guardian immediately requested a meeting with the Facility's Director of Nursing, Executive Director, and Dietitian along with the head chef. She saw to it that Barbara would get healthy meals which included protein in the future!

I received an email from the Guardian a month later. "Our mutual friend" was healing! Her doctors were amazed at the progress she'd made in just four weeks after six months of no progress. Our friend would start using her prosthetic the next week.

Some of you are caring for a friend or family who is living at a Long-Term Care Facility. Like this member, you can still (A)Assess your loved one and be on the lookout for signs of Pain, Infection, Constipation, Environmental Issues, or problems due to a Medication Change. You can also take steps to improve your loved one's care by working with the staff to resolve issues.

Having (G)Gathered important details about the person and (R)Reminisced with them about their past, you now KNOW them. You have also established a (R)Routine that works for them and for you. By knowing the person, establishing a routine, and knowing issues to watch for as you (A)Always Assess, you are now more equipped to preempt or interrupt a behavioral loop!

The next two strategies use the foregoing information. They are to either (C)Calm or (E)Excite a person, depending on the needs discovered.

Sample Medication List

MEDICATION LIST

Name: Susie L. Jones
DOB: 8/19/1945
Updated: 3/21/2021

MEDICATION LIST

Medication Name	Generic for:	Dosage	How many taken?	When Taken	What is it treating?	Prescribed	Date Added or Changed	Notes
Aspirin		81 mg	1 daily	morning	Preventative	Dr. Black	7/1/2018	
Calcium + D3		600/200 mg	1 daily	morning		OTC	9/15/2019	
Cinacalcet	Sensipar	30 mg	1 daily	morning	Alzheimer's	Dr. Black	8/27/2018	
Cranberry + C			2 daily	morning	UTI- Preventative	OTC	1/20/2021	
Donepezil	Aricept	5 mg	1 daily	bedtime	Alzheimer's	Dr. Black	7/1/2018	
Lisinopril	Prinivil	5 mg	1 daily	morning	Blood Pressure	Dr. Black	7/1/2018	Do not give if BP < 100
Melatonin		5 mg	4 daily	bedtime	Sleep Aid	Dr. Black	3/1/2021	
Mirtazapine	Remeron	15 mg	1 daily	bedtime	Alzheimer's	Dr. Black	7/1/2018	
Sertraline	Zoloft	100 mg	1 daily	bedtime	Depression	Dr. Black	7/1/2018	
Stool Softener		100 mg	1 daily	morning	Constipation	OTC	12/15/2020	Give 2 if no BM in past three days
Vitamin B12		1000 TR	1 daily	morning		Dr. Black	8/16/2019	
Zyrtec		10 mg	1 daily	morning	Allergies	OTC	1/18/2021	

Discontinued Medications

Medication Name	Generic for:	Dosage	How many taken?	When Taken	What is it treating?	Prescribed	Date Discontinued	Notes
Omeprazole		40 mg	1 daily		GERD	Dr. Gomez	3/1/2021	no longer needed
Trazodone	Desyrel	500 mg	1/2 daily		Sleep aid	Dr. Black	4/1/2021	caused her to be like a zombie

Dementia with GRACE

Chapter Ten: C for Calm

This falls right in line with the environmental cues from PIC'EM but gets its own chapter because of how particularly important it is to keep overall calm in the atmosphere of someone with dementia. Because their internal life can often be one of low-level anxiety and a general feeling of unease, we need to ensure that their home, room, or care unit is a place of comfort and serenity, as much as possible. We need to become "The Calmest Person in the Room!" I started saying this often in my practice, so it has stuck. I will discuss it now as it relates to the person with dementia, and in the Words of Wisdom section, for caregivers!

(C) CALM is not *just* a description of their environment. Calm is moving from one activity of the day to the next. Having a routine helps with this immensely. If everyone in the person with dementia's environment knows how the day is to go, and there are few disagreements about what is next or where we go next, it keeps down confusion and chaos.

A calm environment looks different for everyone. Your calm might be a beach with crashing waves, whereas another person's calm might be people watching in a busy street-side café. Some people might want more activity in the morning and calming activities at night. (If Sundowning is an issue, this is my recommendation). But some people want to sleep until 10am, slowly ease into their day, and will become more active into the late-night hours. It is a personal preference. Early birds vs. night owls. This preference can last long into the dementia stages. You want to meet the needs of YOUR person.

Needing calm can manifest as rocking, covering their ears, trying to isolate themselves in a corner or refusing to come out of a bedroom, bathroom, or other confining space. It looks like what it is: an overwhelmed person. The behaviors associated with needing calm often present as agitation or aggression. Their internal sense of anxiety is exacerbated by outside noises and chaos, and, in turn, they act out.

In the units I develop for skilled nursing facilities, we have serene murals on the walls, we play Beethoven at breakfast and other soothing music in the dining room throughout the day. We keep the number of residents on the unit low with similar stages of dementia represented.

We make choices which help to maintain peace. There are no overhead intercoms, no ringing phones. We make rules like NO Through Traffic, for instance, so that there is no one on the unit who does not belong, making noise that would otherwise interfere with the quietude of the unit.

We solve for calm, as I say. We think of all possible disruptions to the quiet on the unit and figure out a way to eliminate them. That is not to say that we don't have fun on the unit! We play games and watch movies, have sing-a-longs and enjoy arts and crafts. But we balance that with tranquility. It is a balance, like that flamingo!

In the home, this could be accomplished by having only one TV or radio on at a time. Insisting that people who live in or visit the home maintain a lower level of communication, i.e., NO yelling in the home or otherwise being disruptive. All homes are different, and the population inside them are different. You may be a lady raising three small children and are tasked with also caring for your 88-year-old grandfather with dementia. That is a hard environment to calm! So, you need to be creative with your strategies! But it can be done!

Examples of calming activities include:

- Knitting, crocheting or another needle work
- Tying fishing knots (without the hooks!)
- Coloring (I don't have an issue with any coloring books, but there are adult coloring books now which may be more suited for your person)
- Painting
- Folding clothes (towels are perfect)
- Sorting
- Matching items
- Rocking a baby doll
- Petting a real or plush animal
- Looking at magazines or photo albums

These are just examples of the type of activities that may calm a person to avoid problem behaviors from emerging. You will find, usually through trial and error, what works for your person and what does not.

Remember, failure is a bruise, not a tattoo! If something fails, try the next thing!

Now, some people love the frenzied environment that happens in a house full of noise and competing levels of voices! Again, this is where the G for "Gather Important Details" informs your caregiving. If your person is gregarious and loud and over-the-top, they may enjoy a robust, rousing environment. Loud music, like snappy jazz on the radio, may energize them and meet a need for a more stimulating environment. That is why it is of paramount importance that you get to *really* know your person. It informs all other choices you make in their environment.

Here in the second edition, I am adding the phrase that is probably most associated with me. (It is the most watched video on the YouTube channel) It is this: "Become the calmest person in the room!!"

"HOW?" You may ask...PRACTICE! Practice being calm in traffic, practice being calm in the grocery store, practice with other members of your family. Just practice being calm. And when the time comes to help your person, you can invite them into your calm and not go into their chaos. It's hard, but it can be done.

Just please remember "the broken brain" theory discussed earlier in the book. Their brain is literally dying. That is so hard to hear, but it will make your caregiving go smoother in the reflection of that. "Broken Brain." You wouldn't ask someone with their foot in a cast to run a marathon, would you? Right. So, we cannot expect a mental marathon from a person with dementia.

Chapter Eleven: E for Excite

As some people need calm to maintain their equilibrium and focus, other people need almost constant energizing activity. They need something to **(E) EXCITE** them. If they are too quiet, they get bored; when they get bored, they look for ways to be engaged. If you are not providing for that, they will come up with their own devices. That usually involves wandering, which can then lead to elopement. Not an outcome we want!

Indicators of needing engagement or excitement could be looking around for something to do, pacing, wandering, constantly going to the door or window to look out. They could start looking for their car keys or purse, saying that they must get "somewhere" - to an appointment, to work, to check on something. But they haven't had those responsibilities in quite some time. If they are not able to get up and about, you may see general agitation. They may start vocalizations or asking lots of questions. They *need* engagement. Excitement.

Engaging activities could be a favorite movie from the past. Netflix is great for this! Videos of favorite topics…cooking and baking, dancing couples, adorable kittens, laughing babies…just about any topic has a video on YouTube. With the new TV's these days which connect to the internet, it is easy to "stream" YouTube or Netflix or Hulu or any streaming channel. You can broadcast just about anything! And by engaging them in a video of something interesting to them, you can interrupt a behavioral loop by just turning on the TV!

Similarly, if you know they love to dance, for instance, and you notice them getting fidgety, ask them to dance! Put on some music and cut a rug! This solves the need for engagement AND for exercise, movement or change of position. Even if they cannot stand and dance, you can stand in front of them and use their arms to chair dance.

Most people like to continue to be useful in the home. If you are preparing dinner, give them something to do to help prepare the meal. You will know what they can still do…peel potatoes or make the salad, stir the batter, or tidy up the kitchen while you cook. Certainly, people can still fold clothes, wipe up messes, or dust. Any number of things that will be useful for you and for them. Feeling useful and needed goes a long way to help maintain ego integrity, something we crave as humans.

The main idea is to keep your person as busy *as they would like to be*. If they know they are useful and needed, and making a difference where they are, they will not seek out something to do "out there." If they are made to feel "at home" wherever they are, they will not look for "home" anywhere else. It's a win-win when they can really contribute to the home. Allow them to for as long as they are able.

Chapter Twelve: The GRACE New and Worsening Behavior Tool

Now that you understand the parts of the GRACE Behavioral Management System, let's look at how the parts fit together.

At the end of this chapter, you will find the "GRACE New or Worsening Behaviors Tool" which I developed over almost three decades of working with dementia patients. Working through these steps carefully and in order will help you understand and eliminate or improve problem behaviors. In doing so, you will be helping not only the person with dementia, but you will also be helping yourself by making caring for them a bit easier.

As a caregiver, please keep in mind that these new or worsening behaviors may be as disconcerting to the person you are caring for as they are to you. The person with dementia does not want to be acting ugly or causing problems; their brain is broken. They are not giving *you* a hard time; *they* are having a hard time. Their behavior may be caused by pain, a new or worsening medical condition or infection such as Urinary Tract Infection (commonly referred to as a UTI), an issue with their environment, a medication change, or a number of other factors. It is our job as caregivers to help figure out the causes and solutions of behaviors as quickly as possible - and to help make changes that will eliminate or reduce the behaviors - because the person with dementia can no longer do so for themselves.

So, how do we put the GRACE system into action when a behavior appears?

First, read through the GRACE New or Worsening Behaviors Tool to familiarize yourself with the worksheet found beginning on page 85. Then come back and we'll talk about how to use it. I'll wait right here while you do. Go ahead. Read through all eight pages then we come back here, and I'll explain how to use it.

How to use the New or Worsening Behaviors Tool

When a person with dementia exhibits new or worsening behaviors, a caregiver should walk carefully through the steps of this tool using the GRACE system to determine possible causes or triggers of the behaviors as well as come up with possible solutions.

We will assume that you have been caring for this person for some period of time. You may be caring for them in your home, in their home, or at a long-term care facility. You have noticed a new or worsening behavior. Compared to their behavior a few days or even a few hours ago, something has changed.

You should have used The Gather Tool to (G)Gather Important Information about the person when they first came into your care. A (R)Routine should also have been established. You also have an updated Medication List you can refer to when needed. This list includes the name of the medication, dosage, when it is to be given, and what is treating.

Things were going fairly smoothly. But now, something has changed. What can you do to stop or change the behavior? How can you get Mama to stop doing that??? OR how can you get her to do the thing she is refusing to do??

Before you can resolve the issue, you need to understand the underlying cause of this new or worsening behavior. Before you can "fix the problem" you need to understand what has changed. And you need to discover what may have triggered the change. Remember that these types of issues are often caused by **unmet needs**.

THE ISSUE

You may have noticed the first page of the Tool provides you room to document "The Issue." Documenting exactly what is going on will help you understand, evaluate, and solve the problem. It is also important to write things down not only for other caregivers who may be involved with caring for this person, it will also help medical providers understand what is happening so they may be more able to help you. I find that taking a few minutes to write it all down often helps me see the problem more clearly.

Plus, having this documentation will help you remember what happened, what triggered the behavior this time, and how you solved the issue if it comes up again the future!

(G) GATHER – Quick Look

Quickly think through what you know about this person. Is there something obvious from there past that may be causing the issue? If so, write down quickly. Don't spend too much time on this yet. We will come back to this.

(R) REMINISCE – Quick Look

What from the person's history might help resolve this behavior? Again, this first pass just jot down what you know about their past that might be triggering or leading to this behavior.

(R) ROUTINE – Quick Look

Has their Routine been interrupted? Have family come to visit? Or suddenly stopped visiting? Is there a new caregiver? Has their sleep pattern been interrupted by new activities? Take just a few minutes to think about the Routine.

You may need to contact a family member or any other caregiver to (G)Gather more information about the person or (R)Reminisce to learn more about their history. You may need to adjust the (R)Routine. **But first, you need to (A)Assess them to be sure the cause of this new or worsening behavior is not something requiring immediate medical attention.**

Note: We ALWAYS do Assess first because it is most important. It is the center of **GRACE**.

(A) ASSESS

When a new or worsening behavior appears, the most urgent thing the caregiver should do is (A)Assess the person using PIC'EM. As I said in Chapter Nine, you need to be Always Assessing. Using PIC'EM you need to determine if the person is in P:Pain, has an I:Infection, is C:Constipated, is bothered by the E:Environment, or has had a M:Medication change that may be causing the behavioral change. *Each of these issues except the (E)Environment issues may require immediate medical attention. Especially if the person is behaving a way that may bring harm to themselves or others.*

Carefully work through the steps of PIC'EM on the Tool. Make a check mark by any issues you have noticed. In the space provided, be sure to list any insights you have regarding the signs you are seeing. Write down when you first noticed a symptom, how it is manifesting, and the duration of each occurrence.

For example, if your dad has started moaning when you get him out of bed each day, document anything you have noticed about the moaning? When did you first notice your dad was moaning when you moved him? Does he moan every time you move him or only if you move him to a particular position? Does he seem to be in more pain when he is sitting, standing, or lying down? Have you given him any over-the-counter pain medications? Did they help?

If you see indicators of Pain or Infection including a fever, contact your Home Health Agency or Primary Care provider as soon as you can. Medical intervention may be warranted.

Work carefully through PIC'EM and write out any details and changes you've noticed. Work through ALL the steps as you might find there is a variety of symptoms which may help you and your PCP identify the cause of the change in behavior and together you can work to find a solution.

For example, you may check that you see signs of pain and constipation then notice a new medication was added last week. Could that medication be casing the constipation? Contact your PCP or pharmacist to ask questions.

If your Primary Care Physician makes any medication changes, carefully document the change on the form. Be sure to record the new medication (or the discontinued medication) along with the new dosage. Write our any instructions given by the doctor or pharmacist. You should have a Medication List available to all caregivers. Be sure to update the Medication List to reflect these changes. (There is a sample Medication List in the Appendix.)

(G) GATHER Revisited

Once you have worked through and documented the (A)Assess step using PIC'EM and either eliminated those issues as the cause of the behavior or called for medical care, go back to (G)Gather. Take your time look at the details you have written in your Gather Tool. You may need to call family members or other caregivers to ask if they have any helpful information about why this behavior happened.

(R) REMINISCE Revisited

You may need to sit with your loved one and (R)Reminisce about their life history to help you learn what triggered the behavior. Document what you learn and any actions you take.

(R) ROUTINE Revisited

Look more closely at your (R)Routine. Write out the person's daily routine and scheduled activities. Is it working for you and your loved one? Is too much going on? Not enough stimulation? Are too many people coming in an out? Do you need to change something? Do you need to bring in additional help such as a Home Health Shower Aide? Have you let things slip due to the holidays or vacation? Document what you learn and any ideas you have on correcting the issues. Read Chapter Eight again for ideas on how to set up a Routine for your person.

(C) CALM

As discussed in Chapter Ten, some behaviors happen because the person has become anxious or worried. They may be looking for answers they can no longer remember or reason out. You as their caregiver can help them find the answers they have forgotten or reason out problems they can no longer solve.

You may need to simply talk with them and ask questions. You may need to redirect them to a calming activity such as coloring, knitting, watching a nature video, or looking at pictures of their family.

Document any ideas you have on how to redirect or calm the person. Once you try these ideas, be sure to document the result.

(E) EXCITE

Some behaviors happen because the person is bored or needs to feel like they are needed. Using what you know about the person from your Gather Tool and Reminiscing with them, think of any hobbies or activities they might like to be involved in. What might they be excited to do?

Is there a physical activity you can engage them in? Maybe play their favorite music and get them to sing along or dance with you. Would they do an exercise class with you at the local Senior Center or using a video from YouTube? Do they enjoy gardening? Do they like to do word puzzles?

Were they involved in church choir when they were younger? Could you take them to Choir Practice and let them listen? Ask the choir director if he would be okay with an audience during practice. Maybe they could sit in on the children's choir practices and give the children a round of applause after each song! Or maybe find videos of choirs on YouTube they can watch and sing along with.

For some people folding laundry is always a great option! Keep a stack of clean towels on hand. When she gets bored, unfold the towels put them in a laundry basket, and have them "help you" by folding the laundry.

Some people love to "help" do something. Could you have your dad sort through a bucket of nuts and bolts? Or could your aunt sort through buttons or help color some picture for the neighbor children? Is there a neighbor child that "needs help" with their reading? Could they come over a couple of days to read aloud to your granny?

What might you have your loved one do that they would be excited about? Write out any ideas and try them. Then record the results.

By using this framework, you should be able to IDENTIFY a possible underlying CAUSE of the behavior and use your knowledge of the person to DEVELOP a STRATEGY to solve the behavior issue. Working through these steps will help you manage new or worsening behavior changes.

In the next chapter we will work through a few case studies using this Behavior Tool.

Dementia with GRACE
New or Worsening Behaviors Tool

THE ISSUE

Date it began: _____

Describe the behavior. Include any progression you have noticed.

_____
_____
_____
_____
_____

Who first noticed the issue? How did you first notice it?

_____
_____

How long has this been happening or how often does it happen?

_____
_____

Now that you have identified the Issue, begin to work through GRACE.

Start with a quick look at (G)Gather, (R)Reminisce, and (R)Routine. You will come back and give these a longer look after you have done a complete (A)Assessment. We (A) Assess before an in-depth look at (G)Gather, (R)Reminisce, and (R)Routine because the Assessment may indicate an URGENT MEDICAL issue which needs to be handled

Dementia with GRACE
New or Worsening Behaviors Tool

(G) GATHER – Quick Look

What from The Gather Tool lends insight into the behavior? What do you know about the person from spending time reminiscing with them about their past? This first pass at Gather, just write down what you know about the person that might be impacting or triggering this behavior.

_____
_____

(R) REMINISCE – Quick Look

What from the person's history might help resolve this behavior? Again, this first pass just jot down what you know about their past that might be triggering or leading to this behavior.

_____
_____
_____

(R) ROUTINE - Quick Look

Is a good Routine in place that address the person's general daily schedule at home? Yes/No
Has something happened to interrupt the routine?

_____
_____
_____

(A) ASSESS:

"PIC'EM": Pain, Infection, Constipation, Environment or Medication Change…Issues in ANY of these areas prompt a more thorough medical evaluation and *may* indicate a call to the Physician.

Note: The first step to (A)Assess is to TALK to the person. Ask them if they are in pain. Ask when their last bowel movement was. Ask them if something in the Environment is bothering them. Remember they may no longer be able to verbalize what is going on, but it is still important to talk with them, to communicate with them. Remember to treat them not a problem to be solved but as person to be cared for. While talking with them, WATCH and LOOK for non-verbal signs of Pain, Infection, Constipation, or Environmental Issues.

©2021 Vicky Noland Fitch   Date_____ By:_____

Dementia with GRACE
New or Worsening Behaviors Tool

Nonverbal Indicators of PAIN…check all that apply:

- a look of pain on the person's face
- hand movements that show distress
- guarding a body part or reluctance to move
- moaning with movement
- small range of movement or slow movement
- increased heart rate or blood pressure, or sweating
- restlessness
- crying or distress
- making more or fewer sounds
- withdrawing
- slowness to fall asleep or increased sleep
- disrupted or restless sleep
- low appetite (and consequently low nutritional intake)
- increased confusion
- anger, aggression, irritability or agitation

List any insights and actions taken:
_____
_____
_____

Indicators of INFECTION…check all that apply:

- Frequent urge to urinate (even if the person urinates very little)
- Pain during urination
- Cloudy, red, or strong-smelling urine
- Signs of pain in back, side or lower abdomen
- Nausea or vomiting
- Mental confusion
- Rubbing or pulling on nose, neck or ears
- Tilting or waving head
- Red ears
- Trouble hearing – doesn't respond when called or talked to
- Holding, hitting, or banging head
- Refusing to swallow or eat
- Sounds different from usual (hoarse)
- Earache, fluid coming from the ears
- Sore throat
- Swollen tonsils or lymph nodes
- Bright red throat with white or yellow spots
- Headache
- Stuffy or runny nose
- Pain or pressure in face, tooth pain
- Reduced sense of taste or smell
- Fever – What is their temp? _____

List any insights and actions taken:
_____
_____
_____
_____

©2023 Vicky Noland Fitch   Date: _____ By: _____

Dementia with GRACE
New or Worsening Behaviors Tool

Indicators of CONSTIPATION...Check all that apply:

- Spending a lot of time on the toilet or in the bathroom without explanation
- Straining and grunting while attempting to pass stool
- Refusing to eat or drink
- Hard small and dry feces
- Hard, protruding abdomen
- Vomiting digested food that smells like feces
- Bloating and complaints of stomach discomfort.

List any insights and actions taken:

_____
_____
_____
_____

Indicators of ENVIRONMENTAL ISSUES...Check all that apply:

- Too Hot?
- Too Cold?
- Too Loud?
- Too Busy?
- Too Bright?
- Too Boring?
- Clothes Too Itchy? Too Tight?

List any insights and actions taken:

_____
_____
_____
_____
_____

©2021 Vicky Noland Fitch   Date: _____ By: _____

Dementia with GRACE
New or Worsening Behaviors Tool

MEDICATION CHANGES: Any new medication changes in the last two weeks? Include any over the counter medications, increase or decrease in dosages, etc.

_____
_____
_____
_____
_____

Was the Primary Care Provider contacted? Yes/No

List New Medication Changes:

Medications Added/Increased Dose:

Med Name	New Dose	When given?

Medications Discontinued/Decreased Dose?

Med Name	New Dose	When given?

List any notes or insights including new instructions from the Primary Care Provider:

_____
_____
_____
_____

Have you updated their Medication List? _____

©2021 Vicky Noland Fitch   Date:_____ By:_____

Dementia with GRACE
New or Worsening Behaviors Tool

(G) GATHER

Look through The Gather Tool you filled out when you first began caring for this person. What from The Gather Tool lends insight into the behavior? What do you know about the person from spending time reminiscing with them about their past? You may need to talk to additional caregivers or family members to learn more about the person. What might be impacting or triggering this behavior.

(R) REMINISCE

What from the person's history might help resolve this behavior? Take time to sit and talk with them. Talk to other family members or caregiver. What might be triggering this behavior?

©2023 Vicky Noland Fitch   Date: By:

Dementia with GRACE
New or Worsening Behaviors Tool

(R) ROUTINE

Is a good Routine in place that address the person's general daily routine at home? Yes/No
If not, establish one.
What from The Gather Tool can help you with this routine? For example: Are they an Early Bird or a Night Owl? Do they prefer a morning bath or evening bath?
Write out their routine. Is it working for this person? What adjustments might need to be made?
Is this routine working for the caregivers? Is there some way for the caregivers to adjust to this routine?

(C) CALM:

Does the person need LESS stimulation? What might you do to help calm them?

List insights and actions taken:

© 2021 Vicky Noland Fitch   Date:_____ By:_____

Dementia with GRACE
New or Worsening Behaviors Tool

(E) EXCITE
Does the person need MORE stimulation? What activities might you engage them in?
List insights and actions taken:

_____
_____
_____
_____
_____
_____
_____

RESULTS OF ACTIONS TAKEN

_____
_____
_____
_____
_____
_____
_____

Completed by:
_____

Date: _____ Time: _____

Note:
Keep this form in a notebook or safe place. You may want to refer to it if the behavior starts again or worsens in the future.

©2021 Vicky Noland Fitch   Date:_____ By:_____

How to get a printed copy of the GRACE New or Worsening Behavior Tool

Free Copies of the "GRACE New and Worsening Behaviors Tool" are available in the FORMS section of our Private Group "Dementia with Grace Caregiver Support Group" on Facebook! When prompted with the question "How Did You Hear About Us" answer "The Book"!! We would LOVE to have you join us!

Where to get more help

If you have completed this worksheet, and are still unable to manage the behavior, do not hesitate to contact me at vicky@dementiawithgrace.org so we can brainstorm about what may be happening! I offer reasonably priced 1:1 calls or video conferencing for individual caregivers or all family members, however you want to set it up.

Chapter Thirteen: Examples of the GRACE System at Work

In this chapter, I will take some of the "problem" behaviors we discussed in Chapter Three and give you Real Life examples of this technique at work. These are composites of people and behaviors and situations I have dealt with in practice, and any resemblance of any real person or situation is unintended. I have provided a "GRACE Workup" for each scenario to teach you how I use the tool to identify some ideas and solutions.

Let's dive in!

Pacing: Ralph

Ralph is an 88-year-old retired plumber who loves fixing things. He is widowed, has four children and 12 grandchildren. He has a diagnosis of vascular dementia secondary to a couple of strokes a few years ago; high blood pressure, diabetes, and degenerative joint disease. He lives in the home of his eldest daughter, but all family lives close by. He served in the Air Force, graduated from trade school, and worked as a plumber at a local university for 50 years until his retirement many years ago. After retiring he tended to an award-winning daffodil garden, up until he moved in with his daughter a year ago. He loves to listen to Cole Porter.

Lately, his daughter has noticed that he can't sit still, or won't sit still, for more than a couple of minutes at a time. He is up out of his chair, pacing and puttering and is generally more anxious appearing than at any time previously. He picks up the same picture frames and places them back down, over, and over. He kicks at the rug. He straightens the fern. He checks on the dog bowl. He puts on his coat and takes it off. She says, "Dad, what are you doing", to which is reply is generally, "Nothing, I'm in here." The daughter is afraid he is going to fall. This has been going on now for over a week and she is at a loss as to how to get him just to "sit and rest."

What is happening? Let's figure it out!

Applying the GRACE Behavioral Management System, let's look at some possibilities to help meet his needs.

THE ISSUE

Ralph has become increasingly restless and anxious. He is constantly pacing.

(G) GATHER

His daughter has already (G)Gathered information. I know she has because she told me the information I shared with you!

(R) ROUTINE

His daughter has an established (R)Routine in their home. That has not changed.

We immediately (A)ASSESS Ralph using PIC'EM. *It is important to use PIC'EM early in your evaluation process to rule out any emergent medical issues.* Pain, Infections, Constipation, and Medication Changes are often the cause of sudden behavior changes in people with dementia. As a caregiver, you should ALWAYS be on the lookout – you should ALWAYS be ASSESSING your loved one for signs of medical issues.

(A) ASSESS: "PIC'EM"

> *Pain*: The only non-verbal indicator of pain that we observe is "restlessness", and because he is still able to report pain, we need to ask him if he is hurting anywhere. If so, fix that issue and see if behavior resolves. If not, move on.

Infection: There are no indicators of infection, so we move on.

Constipation: There are no indicators of constipation. Move on.

Environment: He doesn't want to sit still. He is up and about, seemingly looking for things to do. This indicates BOREDOM, i.e.: the environment is too boring. BINGO! Maybe if we solve for boredom, the pacing behavior will resolve!

Medication Change: There has been no medication changes.

Now that we have assessed Ralph and found nothing requiring medical intervention, let's look back at the information we (G)Gathered and see if any of it might help us understand and change the behavior.

(G) GATHER:

We know from both his work history and his after-work history that he probably liked to work with his hands. Being a plumber at a large university probably kept him busy. And after he no longer HAD to work with his hands, he still planted a daffodil garden and tended to it. My guess is that he LOVED to tinker, fix, grow. He loves to listen to Cole Porter.

(R) REMINISCE

He chose daffodils as his plant of choice to tend, experiment with and grow. We can use that preference to find books on daffodils for him to browse; videos on YouTube to watch; or PLANT some daffodils in pots to let him tend. If he can get outside, let him plant in a raised garden or pots. Watch Cole Porter on YouTube if there are any videos available and allow the "Next" video to populate with that same kind of music.

(R) ROUTINE

His daughter may need to adjust the Routine to allow time for Ralph to care for his daffodils or to listen to Cole Porter. For example:

>Rise and Shine!
>Bath/Shower
>Breakfast/Tidy Up Dishes
>Water Daffodils in pots…
>And so forth…

(C) CALM

Boredom, we discovered when evaluating his Environment, was the problem. He didn't need to be Calmed; he needed to be Excited!

Note: Listening to Cole Porter may not be calming; the music may make him want to dance! It might be best to play lively music earlier in the day. Later in the afternoon watching a video on gardening or looking at pictures of flowers – maybe coloring pictures of flowers – would be good choices for late afternoon activities.

(E) EXCITE

Because he is now EXCITED about his daily ROUTINE and his days have meaning once again, his behavior of pacing should resolve!

To review, we used our (A)Assess and ruled out any medical issues, BUT FOUND an environmental issue of BOREDOM, so we used (G)Gather to determine his prior interests, and we used (R)Reminisce and (R Routine to (E)Excite.

Ready to solve another scenario? Good! We have plenty!

Sundowning: Myrtle

Myrtle is a 70-year-old widowed woman who lives in Sunny Side Assisted Living Facility. She has a diagnosis of Alzheimer's dementia, diabetes, and arthritis in her hands. She had no children but has multiple nieces and nephews and their children who visit daily. She is a former nurse. She loves to read, although her reading comprehension does not seem to be what it once was, and her family reports that she will not read a book all the way through anymore. She will, however, watch any movie Liz Taylor stars in.

The staff notes that she is pleasant and cooperative during the day, but toward late afternoon, she seems to become generally more confused and shorter tempered. She wanders away from her room and can be found "looking for my things" in other resident's rooms. This is quite upsetting to the other residents. She will sometimes take off her clothes and look for her "frock" to put on. She has no appetite for supper and is hard to redirect.

What is going on?

Applying the GRACE Behavioral Management System, let's look at some possibilities to help meet her needs.

THE ISSUE

Myrtle gets more confused and shorter tempered in the afternoons. She is wandering and sometimes takes her clothes off. She has no appetite.

(G) GATHER

The staff have gathered information about Myrtle: the know she was nurse and about her family. They know about her medical conditions and her hobbies. There may be more information they can (G)Gather but first they need to Assess her using PIC'EM.

(R) ROUTINE

The facility has an established (R)Routine.

When new or worsening behaviors appear, it is import to (A)Assess the person using PIC'EM early in the evaluation process to rule out any emergent medical issues. Because of her medical conditions, it is especially important that the staff do so with Myrtle! As professional caregivers, they should ALWAYS be ASSESSING their residents for signs of medical issues.

(A) ASSESS: PIC'EM

__Pain__: The only non-verbal indicator of pain that we observe is "restlessness", and because she is still able to report pain, we need to ask her if she is hurting anywhere. When asked, Myrtle says that her "hands ache all the time." Her hands do appear red and swollen. Review of chart reveals that she has diagnosis of arthritis in her hands and does not have any routine pain medicine onboard. A call should be placed to the doctor, and symptoms and complaints reported.

While we are waiting to fix that issue and see if behavior resolves, let's move on can complete the Assessment.

__Infection:__ There are no indicators of infection, so we would move on.

__Constipation:__ The staff reports she has no appetite, which CAN be one indicator of constipation, but we need to look at her appetite. Has her appetite decreased just in the last couple of days? Just at supper? Is the ALF tracking her bowel movements? Or are they depending on her self-report? The goal for an adult is a bowel movement every 3 days. Answer those questions and determine if it *could* be constipation. Solve for that and move on.

__Environment:__ She doesn't want to sit still. She is up and about, seemingly looking "my things." This could indicate *boredom* , i.e.: the environment is too boring. Maybe if we solve for boredom, the behavior will resolve, but it should be noted that this behavior emerges in the *late afternoon* which is indicative of Sundowning.

Medication Change: There has been no medication changes.

(G) GATHER

From Myrtle's history, we know that she was a nurse. We need to dig a little deeper to find out if she was a shift worker, and which shift she worked, not just at the END of her career, but throughout. Because she "will sometimes take off her clothes and look for her 'frock' to put on", that would also indicate that she is getting ready to start a "new" part of her day, i.e., going to work.

The "looking for her things" could be her nurses' bag, her scissors and stethoscope! Provide a bag with those things! Maybe a bag with bandages and a stethoscope (a REAL one, not a pink plastic plaything), and an old blood pressure cuff would appease her when she is worried about her things. It is an easy, cheap fix that just may curb the behavior!

(R) ROUTINE

THIS is what can really help with someone who has an issue with Sundowning. And remember, Sundowning can emerge and resolve over the course of a few weeks or a few months, even if no intervention is found. Even though we are addressing her pain, and looking at whether constipation exists, we can concurrently establish a solid routine which may also help. We know that we can use (R)Routine to lessen the duration and intensity of Sundowning.

Her routine may have been a 3-11 or an 11-7 Work Shift. Ask her! If she is not able to self-report, then the **Gather Tool** will tell us this, hopefully. The daily routine for someone working nights or evenings looks different that someone who worked 7-3.

Ask her if she likes morning baths or evening baths. Ask if she would prefer to sleep late in the morning. (G)Gather all that info, then make a (R)Routine around that data!

If she reports that she likes to sleep late, and always worked a 3-11 shift, her (R)Routine may look like this:

Late morning	Wake Up, Stretch
	Read the Newspaper
	Brunch
Noon	Walk Around the Block
Afternoon	Liz Taylor Movie
Late Afternoon	Snack/Light Lunch… and so forth.

At the above rate, she may want to start her bedtime ritual by getting a good, warm shower around 10:30, after the nightly news. Turning into her bedroom after that with a book. Bedtime may be midnight. And that's ok! It is HER individual routine. It doesn't look exactly like anyone else's!

(C) CALM

The changes in her routine and Liz Taylor albums may calm her.

(E) EXCITE

The nurse's bag and accoutrement should engage her. Talk about the worst patient she ever treated…the funniest, the "miracle" patient. All things nursing which is likely to excite her. Once you get the stories going, she should pick up the thread.

To review, we (A)Assessed her and are contacting the doctor to address her possible pain issue. We will monitor her bowel movements to see if she is constipated. We found a POSSIBLE environmental issue of BOREDOM or SUNDOWNING. We used (G)Gather to determine her prior habits and schedules and (R)Routine to establish a schedule more like it may have once been. We are using the walk in the bright sunlight at noon to stimulate both her body AND her pineal gland. Using (R)Reminisce we have found some Liz Taylor movies to play. And she has her nurse's bag with instruments if she wants to explore that, which should help to (C)Calm her. If she wants to change into her "frock", have a nurse's uniform ready for her to change into. (White shirt/uniform skirt should do). This could also (E)Engage her

Good job! We helped resolve Myrtle's behavior. Should we try another one?

As we discussed in Chapter Three, pacing is different from wandering, which can lead to elopement. Let's discuss them in a person with dementia. We also discussed Ralph's pacing. Next, we will look at the progression from one to another.

Pacing/Wandering which can lead to Elopement: Gertrude

Gertrude is new to this environment, having just moved into her daughter's home. The move was necessary but caused some disruption to the flow of Gertrude's daily routine. The bathroom is in a different place. So is the coffee pot. She has her own suite, with her own furniture; but the chair is not by the window as it was, where she could watch the birds and squirrels with her morning coffee. When she tries to find the chair by the window, it is not there, she has gone back and forth to all the windows, but none of them have chairs. She gets anxious and tries to rearrange some of her things to better suit her and wants to find a chair to sit by the window. She has moved several things in her room, much to the dismay of her daughter, who worked hard to make is a comfortable living environment. There is a window in her room, her daughter tells her, but the furniture looks nicer the way Gertrude's daughter initially arranged it. Gertrude's daughter has so far refused to rearrange the furniture because when visitors come, she wants the room to look a certain way. She is frustrated with her mother scooting furniture around.

Eventually, the pacing and puttering become wandering, as Gertrude moves to different parts of the house looking for her window chair. So, pacing has turned to wandering, especially at night. She has told the daughter that she will just "run out to the store to find a suitable chair", and the family has noticed her trying to leave on a couple of occasions, but so far, she has not left the house. She is determined to find a chair.

Applying the GRACE Behavioral Management System, let's look at some possibilities to help meet her needs. We are meeting needs. Keep that in mind!

THE ISSUE

Gertrude started pacing and rearranging furniture in her room. Then she began wandering throughout the house, especially at night. She is saying she is going to leave! Her family is concerned she is becoming an Elopement Risk.

(G) GATHER, (R) REMINISCE, and (R) ROUTINE

A quick look

We know the move upset Gertrude's (R)Routine. We will come back to that. We will also encourage her daughter to complete The Gather Tool Expanded Edition to help her better understand her mom and to help her know things to (R)Reminisce with her about. But first, we must (A)Assess Gertrude.

We ALWAYS do Assess using PIC'EM first because it is most important. It is the center of GRACE. Using the GRACE Behavior Management System, let's find the unmet need and address this behavior. Remember, (A)Assess is the center of the system.

(A) ASSESS using PIC'EM

__Pain__: The only non-verbal indicator of pain that we observe is "restlessness", and because she is still able to report pain, we need to ask if she is hurting anywhere. If so, meet that need and see if behavior resolves. If not, move on.

__Infection:__ There are no indicators of infection, so we would move on.

__Constipation:__ There are no non-verbal indicators of constipation. Gertrude will not discuss her bowel habits with her daughter. Her daughter may need to keep an eye – or a nose – out to be sure e Gertrude is having regular bowels movements while maintaining Gertrude's wish for privacy in the matter. A change in living conditions often brings with it changes in eating patterns and dietary offerings.

__Environment:__ This is the big red flag in this case. Everything in her environment has changed. This does not require medical intervention, but environmental changes.

Using the PICEM tool we discovered that (E)Environment is the culprit here. In all the ways, make their new space as homelike as possible. (Put a chair by the window!) Maybe have a carafe of hot coffee and a coffee "bar" set up so she can serve herself coffee without the fuss of making a pot, and so that it stays warm all morning.

Although we think we have a solution, we must complete the (A)Assessment and look at any medication changes. Especially since Gertrude is in a new environment with new caregivers. She may have new medications, or her medication regimen may have been disrupted.

Medication Change: There has been no medication changes. Her daughter is diligent to keep her regimen the same as it was before the move since it has been working.

We have assessed Gertrude and found no indictors of (P)Pain, (I)Infection, or (M)Medication Changes. We are fairly sure she is not constipated but have advised her daughter to be aware of symptoms of constipation. We found nothing requiring medical intervention. We are almost certain the (E)Environment is the cause of the wandering. But let's look back at the information we gathered and see if any of it might help us more clearly understand and change the behavior.

(G) GATHER

We see from the Gather Tool her daughter has started that Gertrude loves animals and watching them from inside. She had several bird feeders and plenty of squirrels in her garden to watch. She would spend hours birdwatching.

(R) REMINISCE

Gertrude loves nature and the outdoors. Beyond getting her a chair – which needs to happen TODAY - get some coffee table type books on birds. Or set up a TV in her room where you can play nature documentaries. I'm sure that is not her only interest, the Gather Tool will tell you that, but we know she is missing her chair and birds!

(R) ROUTINE

Gertrude's routine AND environment have changed. I am sure the daughter has set up a beautiful space for her mother, but it is not her home and, it doesn't feel like home yet. Sometimes Gertrude knows they have made the change, for her own good; other times she feels very disconnected to this world. It would be easy enough to set up some bird feeders outside a window and GET A CHAIR for the window!

(C) CALM

Chair by the window!

(E) EXCITE

Chair by the window!

To review, we used our (A)Assess and ruled out any medical issues, but we found an (E)Environmental Issue of her missing a chair by the window. So, we used (G)Gather to determine her prior interests, and (R)Reminisce and (R)Routine to both (C)Calm and (E)Excite!

Sometimes, it can be this simple. Gertrude's daughter had to change HER behavior. The daughter had to loosen up and allow for the guest suite to become her mother's home as much as possible.

Rigidity has no place in the halls of dementia! We must learn to go with the flow!

Shadowing: Juanita

Juanita loves to piddle around her house, rearranging little items and dusting under and around her things. Lately, she has not paid as much attention to her things as she does her husband, Rau. She has started to follow him around incessantly and does not want him out of her sight. He likes to go get coffee in the morning where he meets his buddies. He likes to work out in his workshop. He likes to piddle, too, but by himself. Their marriage has always been smooth, with Juanita doing her things, and Rau; his. But now, Juanita has become his shadow.

Her family has not noticed a functional decline, but Juanita's cognition seems to have slipped more recently. She is misremembering her grandchildren's names. She forgets to shut off the water in the bathroom after washing her hands IF she even remembers to wash her hands. Planning a meal and cooking is beyond her now; Rau has taken over that task. The family is concerned because Rau has started to lose his patience and become aggravated by not having any time to himself.

Using the GRACE Behavior Management System, let's find the unmet need and address this behavior. Remember (A)Assess is the heart of the system.

THE ISSUE

Juanita is declining. She has begun to follow Rau around the house. This constant shadowing is beginning to bother him, causing Rau to lose his patience, and become aggravated.

(G) GATHER, (R) REMINISCE, and (R) ROUTINE

A quick look
We know Juanita is experiencing Cognitive Decline. We will encourage her family to (G)Gather Important Details about her, including her Life History which will help them (R)Reminisce with her as her disease progresses. We will also encourage Rau to establish a (R)Routine. But

first, we must (A)Assess Juanita using PIC'EM to be sure there are issues requiring medical intervention.

It is important to use PIC'EM early in your evaluation process to rule out any emergent medical issues. **As a caregiver, you should ALWAYS be on the lookout – you should ALWAYS be ASSESSING your loved one for signs of medical issues.**

(A) ASSESS using PIC'EM

P: Pain: Juanita is alert and aware enough that she should be able to answer if she is in.

I: Infection: From the review, there is no mention of any signs of infection.

C: Constipation: She may be able to tell you if she is "regular" on her bowel movements.

E: Environment: Nothing has changed in her physical environment. She does seem more needy and wants Rau in sight. She gets anxious when he is not close by. He cannot go to the bathroom alone; she waits for him outside the door. This is an important clue. We will address this in out solution below.

M: Medication Changes: There have been no medication changes.

(G) GATHER

From the Gather Tool, the family reports that this lovely couple has been married for 60 years. They married right out of high school. Juanita has always been a homemaker and loved collecting various things. Her home is filled with mementos and reminders of all the travelling the couple has done over the years. Their children still live nearby. Their children and grandchildren visit regularly. They notice that Juanita's memory is slipping, and she doesn't always call the grandchildren by their names.

(R) REMINISCE

I would suggest here that Rau use her memory of past vacations and adventures to discuss her treasures. She can still tell all about each trinket. Maybe Rau could talk with her about their memories of trips and adventures, using home movies or photo albums.

The family can use this, as well. Perhaps they can schedule a time when the grandchildren come over for a few hours to allow Rau to join his friends at the coffee shop. The grandchildren could record her telling stories prompted by the mementos all around her home. What a treasure that will be to have the provenance of each piece! She is so relaxed and calm discussing her travels.

(R) ROUTINE

Her routine has not changed, except that she is not able to manage her routine on her own. Rau must guide her through her daily routine, reminding her to get a bath (which she can still do), brush her teeth, etc. Breakfast is served and accompanied by him; he no longer goes out to breakfast with his buddies. She can physically do all the things to function independently, but cognitively she must be reminded at almost every step what's next. This is exhausting to Rau. He has tried to go out to the workshop to work on his own projects like he has always done, but he comes back in to find Juanita in an anxious, frightened mood. Once she sees him, however, she is relieved immediately and the anxiety resolves.

(A) ASSESS

The assessment shows us that Juanita is anxious when alone in her home. She is probably straddling the stages between Stage 4 and Stage 5. I would reassure Rau that the behavior she is exhibiting is called Shadowing, which happens right along that time when a person is unsure of situation, time. He is her watch, calendar…compass. If she knows where he is, she knows where she is. It is a powerful connection. A dependency that reassures her.

When she gets deeper into Stage 5, the anxiety will lessen because she "will no longer know what she doesn't know." It is hard on the caregiver to lose more of the person's awareness and connection; but it is easier on the person with dementia. The shadowing does have a natural end, as all behaviors do.

(C) CALM

Right now, Rau needs to focus his energy on meeting this connection need. It will not last forever. Having him close by keeps her calm. In fact, some caregivers in our group report they miss the shadow connection once it resolves.

When he cannot be close to her, he should arrange for someone else to stay with her. Maybe a friend could come over to chat and have coffee every Tuesday or the grandchildren could come over after school on Thursday allowing Rau a few hours each week without his shadow.

(E) EXCITE

Use the Gather Tool to learn all about Juanita. Let her tell her most exciting adventures growing up, their first vacation; the most memorable vacation; a place she never got to visit but wanted to. Look together at travel magazines. Watch videos on YouTube about far away destinations. Meet her need for connection by spending time with her, talking about what she loves to talk about!

Is the GRACE system making sense yet? Let's look at one more example.

Refusing Care/Medicines: Olivia

Olivia is an 89-year-old lady diagnosed with dementia six years ago. She is widowed and has one son. She was an only child and has no other relatives. She lives with him and his wife, which is a recent move. She had been living alone without incident but recently became more confused and needed 24-hour supervision. Lately, she has been refusing her meds, saying that she is being poisoned. She firmly believes her daughter-in-law "wants her dead" and refuses to allow her to provide any type of care. Olivia likewise refuses for the daughter-in-law to come into her bedroom suite; the bedroom and bathroom the couple made suitable for Olivia, should she need to come live with them. There is much tension in the household of three.

Olivia was a homemaker and served on several community projects in her town. She was very active in local politics and was the President of her Homeowners Association for many, many years. She loves to play Bridge, although she can't play well anymore due to concentration and reasoning impairments. Apart from the acrimony with her daughter-in-law, and delusion of being poisoned, she *functions* rather well. She does her own self-care, feeds herself, and performs all other ADLs without issue. Her son doesn't trust her with her medicines because she is on a complicated regimen and wants his wife to administer those for safety. She refuses to take her medicine, and they are at a loss as to how to overcome that resistance. They report she doesn't have any other delusions, hallucinations, or signs/symptoms of psychological distress.

What is going on? This one, I want YOU to try and solve!!

My answers are at the end of the book in Appendix F.

I'll get you started with a few hints on how to proceed.

Read through The GRACE New and Worsening Behaviors Tool in the previous chapter. You will work through the steps as you try to help Olivia's family resolve her problem behaviors. Write down what you observe as you work through the steps. Don't just do them in your head!

Get in the habit of documenting what you found, observed, or discovered as possible causes of the behaviors. List any insights and write what you think should be done to help Olivia.

You may want to make a copy of the Tool or download a full-size copy from the files section of the Dementia with GRACE Caregivers Support Group on Facebook. Of course, you can just use a plain spiral notebook to document your progress through the GRACE steps. Whatever you use, the important thing is to document insights and actions.

Using the Tool, work through the GRACE steps.

Remember to write out the issues. Look at the information above and succinctly write down what the issues are. In the Issues section of the Tool, you don't need to copy ALL the information I gave you.

Then, quickly read through all the information again. What might be included in your (G)Gather Tool for Olivia? (R)Reminisce – think about what you know about her past. Is there a (R)Routine established? Don't spend much time on these steps now; you need to (A)Assess Oliva using PIC'EM.

Work through PIC'EM methodically. Write down any symptoms you she has. Document them from the information I gave you. Is she in Pain? Are there signs of Infection or Constipation? Is there a problem with her Environment? Have there been Medication Changes? If you find any symptoms, document what actions you think need to be taken.

If the (A)Assessment is complete and action has been taken to deal with any medical problems, but behaviors are still present, go back and (G)Gather more information. Do you need to call a family member to learn more? What information that has been Gathered could help you help Olivia?

Look more closely at her (R)Routine. Is there anything that needs to change? Perhaps write out a new Routine this family could implement. Document any insights you gain and actions you think need to be taken.

Look back at the information I gave you. Is there anything that resembles (R)Reminisce: What could you use of this person's history to either help

(C)Calm the behavior or Excite Olivia if boredom is the cause of the behavior?

Now that I've given you hints on what you should do, get to work! Walk through the GRACE steps methodically. Document any insights. Write out how you would solve this family's problems.

Then turn to Appendix F to read my solution and see how you did.

Chapter Fourteen: Words of Wisdom

This chapter highlights phrases or saying which are common to my practice. When you feel discouraged, overwhelmed, or lost, read this chapter!

I have YouTube videos on each of these topics as well. Just go to my channel and search for the title listed after each Word of Wisdom. My YouTube Channel can be found at:

www.youtube.com/c/dementiawithgrace

"Become the calmest person in the room"

This saying is foundational. It is the basis for all caregiving, decision making, interacting.

The broken brain causes a lot of turmoil and chaos, simply because reasoning, insight and judgment are gone. Things just don't make sense. And unlike a growing brain which is learning how to think, a broken, dying brain is forgetting how to think. There are vestiges of knowledge, insight, or reasoning; but it is not complete. It is so frustrating to the person with dementia, especially in those Middle stages of Four and Five. If they come to you for help, and you are equally frustrated; nothing gets accomplished. In fact, you may go backwards or lose ground because now there is more and more frustration, theirs, AND yours. Instead of calm, there is chaos.

You want to invite them into your calm, not descend into their chaos.

But don't you have a right to feel frustrated too? How can you learn to be calm when you feel anything but? Yes, you have every right to feel frustrated, overwhelmed, lost. This is all new to you too. And just when it seems you have strategies figured out, BAM, something new happens that undermines your hard work.

Frustrating!

The difference is this: You have a healthy, intact, working brain. You can read and research. You can reach out for resources, like this book and others, to help you navigate the maze of new feelings, thoughts, and decisions. They look to you.

My strategies? Practice becoming calm in stressful situations that have nothing to do with caregiving. Practice calm in traffic, at the grocery store, online. Give people around you grace to be who they are, not who you need them to be.

Annoying driver tailgating you? Instead of making it about how frustrating it is for you, think of them. Why are they in such a hurry? They don't even know you, so annoying you is not their objective. Yes, they may just be rude, inconsiderate +%&^$s, but they could also be on their way to pick up a sick child from school or late for an important job interview because of a wreck miles up the road you have no clue about. That is where a little grace comes in. And in that grace, calmness. What does that have to do with dementia caregiving? Let's dive into another Word of Wisdom.

"Become the Calmest Person In the Room"

"The person with dementia is not giving YOU a hard time, they are having a hard time."

I'm sure I've said that elsewhere in this book, because I believe that statement to be powerful. It is very rarely about YOU. It being their anger, their aloofness, their accusations, their chaos. It has everything to do with how they are perceiving the world around them; an ever-shrinking world that focuses on their losses and feelings over those losses. I promise you, in most cases, they are not trying to annoy you. They are lost and afraid and need an anchor. A steady hand. Someone who knows what is going on. They do not know they have asked you the same question 25 times. They don't remember the question OR the answer. They just feel confused. You are their touchstone. This is where compassion comes in.

"They Are Not Giving You a Hard Time, They are Having a Hard Time"

"Most behavior is because of an unmet need."

This flows right from the first two words of wisdom: When you are calm and seeing things from the perspective of what they have lost; you can see unmet needs. We have gone into much detail about what these could be: this word of wisdom is to center you back to figuring out that unmet need. In all interactions, but especially when there is a behavior, you need to be Always Assessing. Look at the physical needs of PICEM, but also emotional needs. Are they lonely, frightened, frustrated? Do they want to share something with you that excites them, but they don't have the words? Ferret this out. Calm, compassionate, curious. It all goes hand in hand.

"99% of Dementia Behavior is Due to an Unmet Need"

"Feelings are visitors, not roommates"

This is true for you and for them. Sometimes their feelings change so quickly it makes your head spin! They are frustrated and angry, see ice cream, and all is well! They forget arguments and harshly spoken words rapidly, usually.

For you, however, your intact brain remembers every word…every nuance. You replay it in your mind wondering what you could have said differently. Your memory brings back past hurts and slights. You stew not just in the words of the interaction, but the feelings and memories behind those words. "Maybe I am a bad daughter", you think after the lights go down at night. "Maybe I do treat him like a baby". The feelings of angst and confusion always seem worse at night or when you are alone.

My best advice? Let feelings be visitors. Say, "Hello feeling of condemnation. What are YOU here to teach me?" You may work these feelings out on your own or you may need to seek a qualified therapist. But don't let them unpack in your brain or your soul and move in. It matters how you survive this, do not allow negative, hurtful feelings to define you or your relationship.

"Feelings Are Visitors NOT Roommates"

"All behaviors have a natural end"

Nothing lasts forever, not even demanding dementia behaviors. This word of wisdom is pretty simple, requiring no other explanation. It may take a week, a month, or a stage; but it will pass. And you may even miss it when it's gone. People in the Facebook group often report that they would gladly listen to the same question on repeat just to hear their person's voice again. Sobering thought that informs some of this other wisdom by teaching charity along with calm, compassion, and curiosity.

"What is a Behavior Loop?"

"Home is a feeling, not a place"

This another one of my foundational sayings. Get this right, and you solve the problem of wanting to "go home". Home is a FEELING, not a PLACE. They may be in their own home of 60 years and are asking to go home. You may drive them around to their childhood home, their first married home, or somewhere else you can think of, trying to find "home". You won't find it. You must create it.

Home is family. Home is feeling known. Home is safe. Home is secure. If you can get them talking about what they need to do at "home", who they want to see, etc…it will give you insight into what they are missing. What they NEED. I've said it elsewhere in the book, but I cannot overemphasize how calming it is to feel "known"! When your person with dementia starts asking to go home, dig a little deeper. Meet the need. I have an entire video on this on YouTube, search "I want to go home Dementia with Grace" or go here:

"I Want to Go Home ~Help Calming this Common Dementia Behavior Issue"

"The Power of YES!"

No one likes to hear the word no. It takes away the independence we hold so dear as adults. If you can figure out a way to turn a No into a Yes (or even a maybe), you will buy yourself some time for the behavior to end or morph into one of the interests from the Gather Tool. For instance, "Yes, we can go for another ride but first let's have supper." Then, either do that or depend on the forgetting of car ride by then. Again, full length video on this concept on the YouTube channel!

"How to Fix Behaviors in Dementia with the Power of YES!"

"The Soul Remains"

If being calm is the foundational tool, this is the pinnacle. In every stage, in every dementia, the soul remains. The brain may be broken, the body may fail, but the soul remains.

I believe this with everything I am.

All experiences of a lifetime are not just the facts of a memory but the feelings of the memory. And that is processed in two different areas of the brain. Even deep into Stage 7, a person may not remember who you are, but they can remember the love between you. They know you are someone they love. Soul connections such as smells, music, routines connect us more profoundly than we realize.

"How to Establish Soul Connections"

Chapter Fifteen: You Are a GREAT Caregiver!

Congratulations! You are now even better equipped to continue this long, challenging, rewarding journey as a caregiver! I hope you have found this information useful and will incorporate these tools into your caregiving. Just by virtue of you seeking out MORE information, I know that you are a **great** caregiver!

If you are looking for more knowledge, connection, or insight, I have many ways for you to connect!

> My website: dementiawithgrace.org where you can find links that send you to all my FREE offerings plus ways to work with me one on one!

> Free, Private Facebook Group: "Dementia with Grace Caregiver Support Group" A robust, active support group of others on this same journey. There is SO MUCH information here!

> My YouTube Channel: Dementia with Grace where you will find NEW videos about Caregiver Issues and Difficult Behaviors posted often, with 130+ at time of publishing.

> My email: vicky@dementiawithgrace.org

> Tik-Tok: @dementiawithgrace

I would love to have you connect with us in any way you feel comfortable. You are not alone on this journey.

I want you to remember, there is no PERFECT way to be a caregiver…but there are THOUSANDS of ways to be a **_GREAT_** one!

Wishing you love and joy,

Vicky

One Last Word about GRACE
From the Editor

Three years ago, I began to care for my stepmom who has moderate dementia due to Alzheimer's. I knew practically nothing about caring for a person with dementia. Thankfully, I found "Dementia with Grace" through an internet search. As I read "Dementia with GRACE" and watched Vicky's videos on YouTube, I quickly realized that GRACE is more than an acronym; it is how I should live each day as a caregiver. I must live daily by GRACE. By God's grace.

Grace
(as defined by BlueLetterBible.org)

- that which affords joy, pleasure, delight, sweetness, charm, loveliness: grace of speech
- good will, loving-kindness, favor
- of the merciful kindness by which God, exerting his holy influence upon souls, turns them to Christ, keeps, strengthens, increases them in Christian faith, knowledge, affection, and kindles them to the exercise of the Christian virtues

When caring for a loved one who suffers from dementia, we need God's grace for ourselves. Caring for a person with this disease can be extremely hard at times. We need joy, pleasure, sweetness, and loveliness that comes from Him. We need to have grace from God, so we don't get overwhelmed by the tasks at hand.

As we go through months and even years of caring for a person with Cognitive Decline, we need grace to help us remember that the person with dementia will not get better, will not ever again remember the things they have forgotten, and will continue to lose the ability to do simple things such as feed themselves or use a toilet. As we go through our days of caregiving, we must have grace for the person under our care. We must treat them with dignity, kindness, and gentleness, regardless of how they are behaving.

Yes, some of you are caring for family who were not nice people before their dementia diagnosis. It's hard to be kind to someone who has always treated you poorly or even abusively. It is hard to be gracious to one who has always been mean or selfish. God's grace helps us remember that they are now being impacted by a horrible and frightening disease. They are not in their right mind because their brain is broken. We cannot react to them as if they can control or manage themselves any longer. The disease is destroying their brain. God's grace enables us to care for even these people with kindness, patience, and dignity.

We need grace from and for those around us, including family, friends, and fellow caregivers. We need encouragement. And we need to encourage. We need kindness. And we need to show kind to our fellow caregivers.

We need God's grace and forgiveness when we fail, as we all do at times. We need His grace to remind us that one failure does not mean we are failures. When we fail, we must get up, brush ourselves off, and start again. Sometimes we must apologize to our person, or maybe to others who happened to be in the path of our rage or frustration - maybe a medical provider, nurse, store clerk, or our spouse. We apologize to those we mistreated and ask forgiveness. And we try to do better next time. When you fail in your caregiving, my friend, remember that tomorrow is a new day. Don't let one mess-up get you down. Look up and bask in God's grace. Accept His merciful kindness and let Him exert His holy influence upon your soul.

My friends, I hope this book is as helpful to you as it has been to me as you lovingly care for someone suffering from dementia. And I pray God's grace will strengthen you and guide you in your daily tasks. I pray that in your weak moments you will remember that God's grace is sufficient for you.

Kathleen B. Duncan
Author of "My Journey through Grief into Grace"
and "God's Healing in Grief"

"And he said unto me, My grace is sufficient for thee: for my strength is made perfect in weakness.

"Most gladly therefore will I rather glory in my infirmities, that the power of Christ may rest upon me. Therefore, I take pleasure in infirmities, in reproaches, in necessities, in persecutions, in distresses for Christ's sake: for when I am weak, then am I strong."

2 Corinthians 12:9-10 (KJV)

Notes

Page 2
1. Theses descriptions come from
   https://thekensingtonwhiteplains.com/four-common-types-dementia-2/

Page 4
2. "Genetics of dementia," Alzheimer's Society, December 01, 2016, , accessed June 11, 2017,
   https://www.alzheimers.org.uk/info/20010/risk_factors_and_prevent

Page 5
3. Beason-Held, Lori L. et al. "Changes in Brain Function Occur Years before the Onset of Cognitive Impairment." The Journal of Neuroscience 33.46 (2013): 18008–18014. PMC. Web. 11 Feb. 2018.

4. "10 Early Signs and Symptoms of Alzheimer's ." Know the 10 Signs of Alzheimer's Disease. Accessed June 11, 2017. https://alz.org/10-signs-symptoms-alzheimers-dementia.asp.

Page 9
5. https://www.alzinfo.org/understand-alzheimers/clinical-stages-of-alzheimers/

Page 11
6. https://www.pbm.va.gov/PBM/clinicalguidance/drugmonitoring/FunctionalAssessmentStagingFAST73108.doc

Page 20
7. https://www.alz.org/care/dementia-medic-alert-safe-return.asp

Page 45
8. Eifler, Amy. 1997. The DETA brain series. [Tuscaloosa, Ala.]: University of Alabama Center for Public Television & Radio.

Page 50
9. López-Muñoz F., Marín F., Álamo C. (2016) History of Pineal Gland as Neuroendocrine Organ and the Discovery of Melatonin. In: López-Muñoz F., Srinivasan V., de Berardis D., Álamo C., Kato T. (eds) Melatonin, Neuroprotective Agents and Antidepressant Therapy. Springer, New Delhi

APPENDIX

Appendix A: 10 Signs and Symptoms of Alzheimer's

1. MEMORY LOSS THAT DISRUPTS DAILY LIFE
2. CHALLENGES IN PLANNING OR SOLVING PROBLEMS
3. DIFFICULTY COMPLETING FAMILIAR TASKS AT HOME, AT WORK OR AT LEISURE
4. CONFUSION WITH TIME OR PLACE
5. TROUBLE UNDERSTANDING VISUAL IMAGES AND SPATIAL RELATIONSHIPS
6. NEW PROBLEMS WITH WORDS IN SPEAKING OR WRITING
7. MISPLACING THINGS AND LOSING THE ABILITY TO RETRACE STEPS
8. DECREASED OR POOR JUDGMENT
9. WITHDRAWAL FROM WORK OR SOCIAL ACTIVITIES
10. CHANGES IN MOOD AND PERSONALITY

From : "10 Early Signs and Symptoms of Alzheimer's ." Know the 10 Signs of Alzheimer's Disease. Accessed June 11, 2017. https://alz.org/10-signs-symptoms-alzheimers-dementia.asp.

Appendix B: Seven Stages of Dementia

The Seven Stages is vernacular for the Global Deterioration Scale (GDS).

Stage 1: No Impairment
During this stage, Alzheimer's is not detectable, and no memory problems or other symptoms of dementia are evident.

Stage 2: Very Mild Decline
The senior may notice minor memory problems or lose things around the house, although not to the point where the memory loss can easily be distinguished from normal age-related memory loss. The person will still do well on memory tests and the disease is unlikely to be detected by loved ones or physicians.

Stage 3: Mild Decline
At this stage, the family members and friends of the senior may begin to notice cognitive problems. Performance on memory tests is affected and physicians will be able to detect impaired cognitive function.

People in stage 3 will have difficulty in many areas including:
Finding the right word during conversations
Organizing and planning
Remembering names of new acquaintances
People with stage three Alzheimer's may also frequently lose personal possessions, including valuables.

Stage 4: Moderate Decline
In stage four of Alzheimer's, clear-cut symptoms of the disease are apparent. People with stage four of Alzheimer's:
Have difficulty with simple arithmetic.
Have poor short-term memory (may not recall what they ate for breakfast, for example)
Inability to manage finance and pay bills.
May forget details about their life histories.

Stage 5: Moderately Severe Decline
During the fifth stage of Alzheimer's, people begin to need help with many day-to-day activities. People in stage five of the disease may experience:
Difficulty dressing appropriately.
Inability to recall simple details about themselves such as their own phone number.
Significant confusion
On the other hand, people in stage five maintain functionality. They typically can still bathe and toilet independently. They also usually still know their family members and some detail about their personal histories, especially their childhood and youth.

Stage 6: Severe Decline
People with the sixth stage of Alzheimer's need constant supervision and frequently require professional care. Symptoms include:

Confusion or unawareness of environment and surroundings
Inability to recognize faces except for the closest friends and relatives.
Inability to remember most details of personal history.
Loss of bladder and bowel control
Major personality changes and potential behavior problems
The need for assistance with activities of daily living such as toileting and bathing
Wandering

Stages 7: Very Severe Decline
Stage seven is the final stage of Alzheimer's. Because the disease is a terminal illness, people in stage seven are nearing death. In stage seven of the disease, people lose the ability to communicate or respond to their environment. While they may still be able to utter words and phrases, they have no insight into their condition and need assistance with all activities of daily living. In the final stages of Alzheimer's, people may lose their ability to swallow.

From: https://www.alzinfo.org/understand-alzheimers/clinical-stages-of-alzheimers/

Appendix C: Terminology and Abbreviations

ADL – Activities of Daily Living

Age in Place – Refers to a person continuing to live in a facility even as their dementia progresses. Some facilities allow residents to Age in Place through hospice and until death.

ALF – Assisted Living Facility

Behavioral Loop - The beginning of a behavior problem to its natural end.

CNA – Certified Nursing Assistants

DON – Director of Nursing

Gather Tool – Document used to gather important details a person including their Life History

HHA – Home Health Aide. Also called Personal Care Aide

HHC – Home Health Care

Life History – Information to be gathered about a person's past

LBD – Lewy Body Dementia

LO – Loved One

LPN-Licensed Practical Nurse

LVN – Licensed Vocational Nurse

MC – Memory Care Unit

MCI – Mild Cognitive Impairment

MCU – Memory Care Unit

Medication List – A list of all medications a person is taking including details about each one.

NH – Nursing Home. Also called a Skilled Nursing Facility

PCA – Personal Care Aide. Also called Home Health Aide

PCP – Primary Care Provider

PRN – Medical term for "As Needed" used often for medications. Example: 1 Tablet PRN means take 1 tablet as needed.

PWD – Person with Dementia

Resident – Person living in a facility

RN – Registered Nurse

SNF – Skilled Nursing Facility. Commonly referred to as a Nursing Home

UTI – Urinary Tract Infection

UA – Urinary Analysis, a test to detect a UTI

UA C & S – Urinary Analysis with Culture and Sensitivity

Appendix D: GRACE

G: Gather Important Details

R: Reminisce/Routine

A: Always Assess (PIC'EM)

    P: Pain
    I: Infection
    C: Constipation
    E: Environment
    M: Med Change

C: Calm

E: Excite

Appendix E: The GATHER Tool

Instructions for Use:

Completing this document is the first step in the GRACE Behavior Management System to "Gather Important Details." It sets the foundation of everything else to follow. Know that the information you Gather using this tool will be invaluable to making sure the other components work. Knowing the answers to these questions will inform how you interact with the person with dementia. For instance, knowing a person's favorite type of music, and LEAST favorite could help calm them OR engage them, depending on the behavior you are managing.

I would suggest reading through the questionnaire first to become familiar with the questions. Some might not be appropriate or needed. This is a good guide, but feel free to add or subtract from it as you see fit!

You will know best how to ask the questions to your loved one. Some people will welcome these questions exactly as they are presented here, with you jotting down the answers as you go. Some people would answer more readily if the questions were presented in a conversational style, a few at a time. Some loved ones would be VERY suspicious if you took out a pen and started writing down anything they said. Others would welcome the attention and focus on their lives.

It is a very personal exercise, and you should be respectful of their feelings, attitudes, and answers. If your loved one does not want to answer a particular question or delve deeper into a subject, respect that. Also, make a note of where an issue surfaced. That can be informative, too. For instance, if they are answering questions just fine, but clam up when military service is mentioned, that could indicate an underlying issue in that area. It might inform you not to bring up that subject again, or it may give insight into a behavior down the road. Similarly, highlight any information that makes a person "light up"! An area on which they could talk for hours! This will be your "go-to" topic to distract them if a behavior loop emerges!

All information, verbal and non-verbal, is helpful when dealing with someone with dementia. There will come a time when they are no longer able to answer these questions, and the information you gather while they ARE able will provide you a road map for when they are not.

Of note, if you are at a stage with your loved one where they are no longer able to answer these questions; use your own knowledge of their past to help flesh out the information or ask siblings or friends.

And lastly, have fun! Use these questions as a guideline. If a neat story comes up, go with it! You may learn more than you would have if you just skipped to the next question just for the sake of it! Engage in a conversation with your loved one; answer the questions yourself along with them! There is no right or wrong way to do this, so just jump in and see how it goes!

I suggest that this tool be kept with the person across the continuum of care. New caregivers or sitters in the home, temporary caregivers in a hospital setting, and caregivers in a new facility, should your loved one require that level of care. Of course, a copy of this book with how to use the tool and the supporting steps would be a useful resource, as well.

An expanded version of the Gather Tool is coming in summer of 2021. The workbook will be titled, "The GRACE Gather Tool (Expanded Edition)" and will be available for purchase through online bookstores.

Name:

What is your full name? (First, Middle, Maiden, Last)

Who named you?

Were you named after anyone in particular? Why?

Do you have any nicknames?

Who gave you a nickname? Why? What does it stand for?

Have you ever gone by any other names? Another married name? Another first name?

What are you called by your spouse? Children? Grandchildren? Siblings?

What do you prefer to be called?

Childhood Memories:

Where were you born? What town/city/state?

Were you born in a hospital? At home?

Who were your parents? (Names)

What did you call them? (Mama, Papa? Mother, Father?)

What kinds of jobs did they have?

Did you have any brothers or sisters?

What are their names?

Did you have any nicknames for them?

Are you the oldest, youngest? Where do you fit in the family?

What is your earliest memory from childhood?

Tell me about your home...

Did you have any pets?

Did you grow up in the city? On a farm? In a big place or small?

Tell me about your neighborhood...

Who were your best friends growing up? Tell me something about them...

Where did you go to school?

What was your favorite thing about school?

What was your best subject? Worst subject?

Tell me about your teachers...

What did you want to be when you grew up?

Did you have any role models or heroes as a child? Who did you look up to?

What fascinated you as a child? What did you like to study or talk about?

What new inventions did you like the most? Cars? Television? Space travel?

Tell me how you spent your time as a child...

Adulthood:

Were you ever married?

Who did you marry?

How did you meet your spouse?

How did you propose/how were you proposed to?

How long have you been married?

Tell me about your wedding...

Did you have any children?

What are their names?

Any grandchildren? Names...

Tell me about your children...

Education and Work History:

Did you go to school to study a trade?

Did you go to university or college?

Did you ever serve in the military?

How did you decide what to do after high school?

What was your first job?

What was your main job or career in your life? Did you enjoy your work?

Tell me what you liked most about your job? Least?

Hobbies:

What do you like to do for fun?

Do you like to play games? Read? Write? Draw? Sing? Cook? Etc...

What do you like to read? Magazines? Fiction? Biographies? Religion?

What are your favorite things to watch on TV?

Any favorite movies?

Where do you like to go on vacation?

Tell me about some of your favorite vacations...

What are some of your favorite foods? Least favorite?

If you could travel anywhere in the world, where would you go?

If you could talk to anyone in the world, who would you talk to?

If money were no object, what would you buy?

Miscellaneous:

Favorite color?

Favorite song?

Favorite actor?

Favorite food?

Favorite actress/actor?

Favorite movie star?

Favorite singer?

Favorite type of music?

Favorite car?

Favorite place to spend time?

The Gather Tool

Additional copies of the Gather Tool are available online. Join our Private Facebook Group "Dementia with Grace" and look in the Files sections. When prompted with the questions "How Did You Hear About Us,' answer "The Book"!! We would LOVE to have you join us!

An expanded version of the Gather Tool is coming in summer of 2021. The workbook will be titled, "The GRACE Gather Tool (Expanded Edition)" and will be available for purchase through online bookstores.

Appendix F: Solution for Olivia

THE ISSUE

Olivia refuses to take her medications. She believes she is being poisoned by her daughter-in-law.

(G) GATHER INFORMATION

Her daughter-in-law has gathered important information, which we will come back to.

(R) REMINISCE

We know she was a homemaker and active in her community. We may need to think about these.

(R) ROUTINE

There does not seem to be an established Routine in the home. We will work on that, but, first, we need to Assess Olivia to decide if there is a need for medical intervention.

(A) ASSESS: PIC'EM

Pain: There are no verbal OR non-verbal indicators of pain based on what we know, so let's move on.

Infection: There are no indicators of infection, so we would move on.

Constipation: There are no indicators of constipation, so we move on.

Environment: Olivia stays in her room, self-isolating from the new environment she is in. I see from her "Gather" info that she was a very active homemaker, to the point of taking on the responsibility of governing her whole Homeowners Association committee! That is dedication to your living environment and surroundings! She also liked to play Bridge, which was a weekly social outlet for her. Isolation can allow her to sit there with her mind free to "speculate" about her circumstances, and if she is sad, angry, or otherwise upset about having to leave her home and go into a home where she has no authority, these feelings can fester. Her "broken brain", assaulted by dementia, may then conflate her feelings of anxiety and agitation, and come to the faulty conclusion that her daughter-in-law wants to harm her (she thinks THAT is why she feels anxious), and continues that line of thinking to assume then that she is being poisoned. Her brain is playing tricks on her. Because of this, she now refuses for her daughter-in-law to even come into the room.

Medication Change: She is on a "complicated regimen" of medicines according to son. The doctor should be made aware of her refusal, and an assessment should be made to see if ANY of that medicine be consolidated or changed. Sometimes, people have not had a GOOD review of their medicines after even YEARS of being on the same routine. A good, thorough review can be conducted at an appointment with her PCP to see if fewer meds can be given, or if any of them could be accomplished in a single dose, verses multiple doses. Can ALL medicine be given at a single medicine pass? Or somehow otherwise simplified. ALSO, he may decide that a psychotropic medication is needed to address the delusions. The doctor and his nurse should be more than happy to help with this aspect of the solution.

While waiting on a returned call from the Primary Care Provider regarding medication changes, let's look back at the information gathered and see how that may help us.

(G) GATHER

We know from her Life History that she is an only child. She also was incredibly involved in local organizations at the leadership level. This indicates to me that she has probably always been a leader, not a follower, and that she is accustomed to things happening because of her, not things happening TO her. She probably feels vulnerable being "TAKEN care of" when SHE has always been the one "TAKING care of." Does that make sense? She was always in control, in one way or another, of herself, her home, her community. Now, the tables have turned, and she is no longer in complete control. We need to figure out how to give control back to her, in ALL the ways that we can. Once the medicine is sorted out, one thing to do would be to give her control once again of a very simplified routine. For example, if she has multiple pills, put one in each slot of a medicine organizer, and allow her to take one pill at a time, on her own, and YOU supervise if all the pills were taken. It will take more time, but the goal is to get the medicines down!

(R) REMINISCE

Bridge was such a part of her life at one time, I would try and get her active in that again. Maybe "teach" the daughter-in-law to play!! That would put her in a "power position" over the daughter-in-law and may very well balance the dynamic. Buy some books on beginning bridge and have the daughter-in-law ask her "opinion" on the books. More than likely, she will assert that she "knows more than those silly books" and offer to become the expert for her! Even if she can't play OR teach very well, it is the "power" balance that is reestablished that can make the difference in her behavior!

(R) ROUTINE

Set a daily Routine for her medicine. Same time, same place, same way. Make no argument, present the medicine as "the next thing" after breakfast, lunch…whatever. Connect it with something she WILL do, and have it naturally flow as the next item to do.

(C) CALM or (E) EXCITE

In this scenario, she needs calming more than exciting. Having her medicines simplified, her power reestablished in the mother/daughter-in-law scenario, and the reengagement into bridge; hopefully, her mind will be settled that she is loved and cared for, has power, and is in some control of her life once again.

To review, we used our **(A)Assess** and found a need to simplify her medicines, and an environmental issue of self-isolation and possible boredom, as well as a loss of power and choice component. A need for autonomy. We used **G)Gather** to determine her prior interests, and **(R)Reminisce** and **(R) Routine** to **(C)Calm**.

How did you do? If you have ANY questions with this exercise, visit www.dementiawithgrace.org for ways to connect with me and get more intensive training!

Thank you for buying my book! I hope it helps! See you in the group soon!

Vicky

Appendix G: Sample Medication List

MEDICATION LIST

Name: Susie L. Jones
DOB: 8/19/1945
Updated: 3/21/2021

Medication Name	Generic for:	Dosage	How many taken?	When Taken	What is it treating?	Prescribed	Date Added or Changed	Notes
Aspirin		81 mg	1 daily	morning	Preventative	Dr. Black	7/1/2018	
Calcium + D3		600/200 mg	1 daily	morning		OTC	9/15/2019	
Cinacalet	Sensipar	30 mg	1 daily	morning	Alzheimer's	Dr. Black	8/27/2018	
Cranberry + C			2 daily	morning	UTI- Preventative	OTC	1/20/2021	
Donepezil	Aricept	5 mg	1 daily	bedtime	Alzheimer's	Dr. Black	7/1/2018	
Lisinopril	Prinivil	5 mg	1 daily	morning	Blood Pressure	Dr. Black	7/1/2018	Do not give if BP < 100
Melatonin		5 mg	4 daily	bedtime	Sleep Aid	Dr. Black	3/1/2021	
Mirtazapine	Remeron	15 mg	1 daily	bedtime	Alzheimer's	Dr. Black	7/1/2018	
Sertraline	Zoloft	100 mg	1 daily	bedtime	Depression	Dr. Black	7/1/2018	
Stool Softener		100 mg	1 daily	morning	Constipation	OTC	12/15/2020	Give 2 if no BM in past three days
Vitamin B12		1000 TR	1 daily	morning		Dr. Black	8/16/2019	
Zyrtec		10 mg	1 daily	morning	Allergies	OTC	1/18/2021	

Discontinued Medications

Medication Name	Generic for:	Dosage	How many taken?	When Taken	What is it treating?	Prescribed	Date Discontinued	Notes
Omeprazole		40 mg	1 daily		GERD	Dr. Gomez	3/1/2021	no longer needed
Trazodone	Desyrel	500 mg	1/2 daily		Sleep aid	Dr. Black	4/1/2021	caused her to be like a zombie

About the Author

Vicky Noland Fitch is a social worker and dementia consultant with a Bachelor of Science degree in Social Work (BSW) from the University of Montevallo. She is also a Certified Dementia Practitioner (CDP). She has worked for almost three decades in long term care serving the elderly population and their families. She has developed the framework, structure and programming for multiple memory care units, and the behavior management systems they employ. She actively consults with families and facilities; educates and trains caregivers, writes about her failures and successes in caregiving, and talks about dementia to any willing audience.

Vicky has a deep desire to understand dementia more fully, so she can translate that knowledge into helping people with dementia and their caregivers, both personally and professionally.

Vicky is a small-town girl who lives and works out of an 1892 farmhouse in Alabama. She may be reached at vicky@dementiawithgrace.org

Contact the Author

Vicky Noland Fitch

Dementia with GRACE Facebook Page:
www.facebook.com/dementiawithgrace

Dementia with Grace Facebook Support Group:
www.facebook.com/groups/dementiawithgrace

Vicky's Email: vicky@dementiawithgrace.org

YouTube: youtube.com/c/dementiawithgrace

Tik-tok: @dementiawithgrace

Amazon Store:
www.amazon.com/store/dementiawithgrace

Website: dementiawithgrace.org

Made in the USA
Columbia, SC
05 October 2023